D0108996

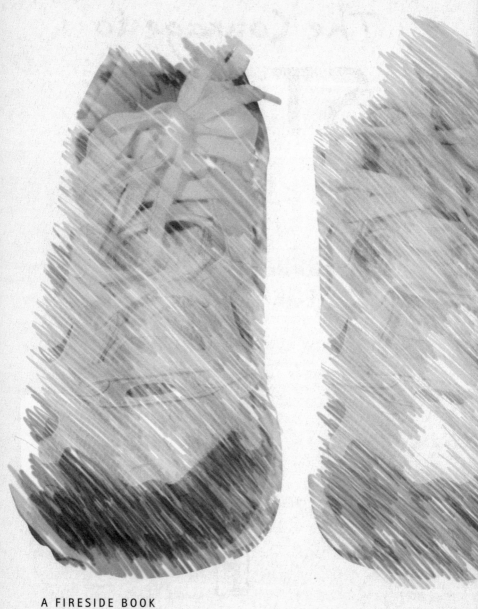

A FIRESIDE BOOK

SIMON & SCHUSTER

The Courage to
START

A GUIDE TO RUNNING
FOR YOUR LIFE

John "THE PENGUIN" Bingham

FIRESIDE
Rockefeller Center
1230 Avenue of the Americas
New York, NY 10020

FIRESIDE and colophon are registered trademarks
of Simon & Schuster Inc.

Designed by Maura Fadden Rosenthal/Mspace

Manufactured in the United States of America

10   9   8   7   6   5   4   3   2

Library of Congress Cataloging-in-Publication Data

Bingham, John, 1948–
      The courage to start : a guide to running for your life / John
   "The Penguin" Bingham.
         p.   cm.
      Includes index.
      1. Running.   2. Running—Psychological aspects.   I. Title.
   GV1061.B55   1999
   796.42—dc21
                                                      99-17797
                                                        CIP

ISBN 0-684-85455-4

To Mart,
for all the miles
you never got to run

ACKNOWLEDGMENTS

I like to read acknowledgments. I'll read the acknowledgments even if I have no intention of buying the book. I may not find out much about the book, but I find out a lot about the author: whether they think they got to where they are by themselves (I don't), and whether they recognize how truly fortunate they are that they got to put their thoughts and feelings into print (I do).

My entire life has been an apprenticeship for this moment, and to thank all those who have taught me, gently or harshly, would look like a biography. There are those who believed in this project long before I did and others who withheld their support to protect themselves in case it failed. I am grateful to the believers for helping me start and to the doubters for giving me the incentive to finish, if only to prove them wrong.

It all begins with family, and there I have been lucky. The struggle to find oneself is made easier if you have the light of love. Many of those who have been the brightest lights are not here to read the words, but my life stands as testimony to their caring. To those who are here, to my mom and dad and my brother, I send my gratitude.

I want to thank my son, Terry, especially, for showing me in himself the best of everything I ever hoped for in myself. If it is true that the child is father to the man, then he is surely the finest teacher I have ever had.

There are more recent mentors and friends, who, although they have seen only the most current me, are nonetheless important contributors to who I am becoming. There is Marlene Cimons, who saw something in my words, and Nicole Brodeur, who first put the process of me becoming myself into writing. Thank you.

I want to thank Amby Burfoot, executive editor of *Runner's World* magazine, for having the courage to publish the first "Penguin Chronicle," and Mark Will-Weber, whose editing of those columns made them better than I had ever dreamed they could be.

Thanks also to Sue Flaster, who sat through hundreds of pancake breakfasts listening to me panic, and Linda Roghaar, who dragged me around New York City like a wet puppy.

And, of course, my thanks go out to the thousands of runners who have allowed me to look inside their lives. In particular, I want to thank the most wonderfully strange group of people who are members of the Penguin Brigade. This extended virtual family proves to me that there will always be a reason to believe in tomorrow.

Finally, I would like to thank my wife and running partner, Karen, for the countless hours she has invested in this book and for the years she has invested in me. With every step we run, we discover each other and ourselves.

Without her, none of this would have been possible. And, more to the point, without her, becoming myself wouldn't have been worth the struggle.

CONTENTS

Part Three: The Road to Victory

Part Four: Running for Your Life

INTRODUCTION

As a child I loved to run. Looking back, I think I ran almost all of the time. I loved the feeling of moving from where I was to where I wanted to be. When there was no reason to run, I ran anyway. I liked games in which you had to run. I ran when I should have, and I ran when I shouldn't have. I ran into things, and over things, and around things.

Then, one day when I was nine or ten years old, I found out that I wasn't any good at running. I was shocked. It wasn't that I was just a little slower than other kids. I really wasn't any good at all. My legs went in all the wrong directions, my arms flailed, my feet flipped and flopped. I stank.

What made me so sure? Easy. Everyone told me so. Friends told me. Teachers told me. Coaches told me. And I told myself. I found out that almost everyone I knew was faster than me. From that moment on, I wasn't running, I was chasing.

Chasing isn't nearly as much fun as running. Being last, always last, stopped being fun almost immediately. Despite the joy that I had experienced in running as a child, by the middle of my elementary school years I was convinced I would never be an athlete.

Participating in team sports only added to my childhood pain and frustration. I was always last there, too. Have you ever been the last one picked to be on a team? Have you ever had the humiliating experience of watching as everyone but you is chosen? I did. Often. I was picked to be on the team as an afterthought. Not so much because I had been chosen, but because there was no one else left to choose.

So I stopped running for nearly forty years. Though nothing was as satisfying as running, I found other activities that interested me. It would be kind to call those activities hobbies. They weren't. They were places to hide. They were substitutes for the activity I missed the most. Running. Like many other people, I fooled myself into thinking that if I was successful at my job or had bigger houses and faster cars, I would forget the pain of being picked last. I didn't forget. You probably haven't either.

So, as an adult, I missed the joy of moving my body. I spent nearly all of my leisure time watching other athletes do what I thought I could not do. I watched them run. I watched them play football and baseball and race motorcycles. I dreamed that I was one of them. I was not alone. Every weekend stadiums and living rooms are filled with people like me, people who believe that living the life of an athlete vicariously is as good as being an athlete yourself. It isn't.

It was a mistake to quit running. I know that now. It was a mistake to give up the joy I felt when I moved my body with nothing more than my own legs, to let others steal my satisfaction from me. It was a mistake I won't make again.

At age forty-three, when I decided to run again, I realized that the images used to describe runners didn't fit me. I wasn't a rabbit. I wasn't a gazelle or a cheetah or any of the other animals that run fast and free. But I wasn't a turtle or a snail either. I wasn't content anymore to move slowly through my life and hide in my shell when I was scared.

I was a round little man with a heavy heart but a hopeful spirit. I didn't really run, or even jog. I waddled. I was a Penguin. That was the image that fit. Emperor-proud, I stand tall to face the elements of my life. Yes, I am round. Yes, I am slow. Yes, I run as though my legs are tied together at the knees. But I am running. And that is all that matters.

As I have told my story, I have discovered that there are Penguins everywhere. They are the runners you see in your neighborhood. They are the runners who race without hope of winning. If you are a fast runner, the Penguins are the ones who are still on the race course when you are driving home.

Rediscovering the simple pleasure of running as an adult is a strange, frustrating, wonderful, confusing, and ultimately immensely satisfying preoccupation. It's hard to erase all the old images of yourself as clumsy and uncoordinated and forget the feeling of isolation you felt when you were always the last one chosen.

But it can be done. You can go from a 240-pound couch potato to a 150-pound marathoner. You can overcome addiction and drug or alcohol abuse. You can overcome a lifetime of failing. It takes a little time for most of us, but thousands of runners who have no more reason to succeed than you do have done it. I did it. They did it. You can, too.

Successful "adult-onset" athletes are made, not born. To those of us who simply want to run, the value of genetics is highly overrated. Running doesn't require an extraordinary combination of muscle and bone. It requires only the desire to move our bodies and the wisdom to accept the difference between our will and our won't.

Running, like living, is alternately easy and hard, good and bad, exciting and boring. It is made up of long periods of dreadful sameness interrupted by brief moments of pure exhilaration. The big difference between running and life is that runners can choose their moments of exhilaration.

Those moments are available to us every time we put on our running shoes. The highs and lows of a lifetime can be experienced in a single run or race. From anticipation to letdown, from abject terror to unbridled happiness, the emotions of living are there at every foot strike.

Runners may not be any more honest than the rest of the population, but I think they are. You can pretend to be smart or wealthy.

You can rent a lifestyle for a week. For a few hours or a few days, you can deceive those around you, and for a while, yourself.

But as a runner, you have to face the truth about yourself on a regular basis, and it makes you more honest. You can't pretend to be faster than you are. You can't pretend that you are better prepared than you are. You cannot pretend to be a runner, you actually have to run.

In the end, being a runner is no more complicated than that. To be a runner, you simply have to run. It's not enough to dream about being a runner. It's not enough to plan on being a runner. Sooner or later, you have to run.

And if you run, you are a runner. It doesn't matter how fast or how far. It doesn't matter if today is your first day or if you've been running for twenty years. There is no test to pass, no license to earn, no membership card to get. You just run.

Some time ago, I wrote a column for *Runner's World* magazine about putting action into your dreams. I was watching a young boy, alone on an empty baseball field, who kept swinging an imaginary bat until he hit an imaginary home run. At that point he put his dreams into action. He ran around the bases.

My mother, who became an athlete at the age of sixty-four, is a great supporter but honest critic of mine. She hated that column. She focused on the boy *before* he hit the home run. She said she felt sad for him because he was there alone. Sad because there was no one for him to play with, no one with whom he could share his dream.

I tried unsuccessfully to explain to my mom that she had missed the point. The point wasn't that the boy was alone. The point was that despite the fact that he was alone, he lived out his dream and celebrated his home run.

We all need to live out our dreams. We need to spend less time planning and organizing and more time doing. We need to spend less time worrying about doing things well and more time rejoicing that we are doing them at all.

The real joy begins when we, like that boy, run the bases. The celebration begins when we stop deciding if we are going to run or how we are going to run, and start deciding *when* we are going to run. The miracle begins by taking the first step.

The Courage to Start shows how, with that first step and with every subsequent step, you can begin to write your own story. It shows how each of us, no matter how ordinary we may seem, is capable of greatness . . . if we will only risk starting.

What you will read in this book is just about everything I know about running and just about everything I know about myself. It's everything I have learned, everything I have been told, and every discovery I have made. There are no secrets. It is just you and me . . . and the road that we are on.

That road is not always smooth or flat. There are times when it may seem as though you are running away from who you are much more than running toward who you want to be. There may be times when your body betrays you and your spirit abandons you. The path to enlightenment is not always clearly marked.

But millions of runners have gone before you. Each of them has faced the same fear and uncertainty. Each has learned, as you will, the truth in the Penguin credo. For all of us, the miracle isn't that we finish, the miracle is that we have the courage to start.

Part One

THE COURAGE TO START

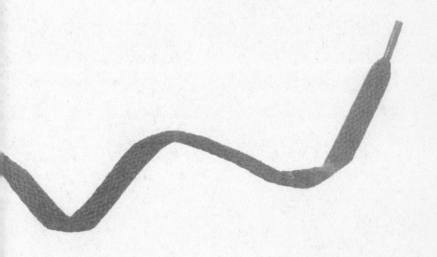

1

The Courage to Start

Every January it was the same story. Like so many others I looked to the New Year as the time to start my new life. I started thinking about it in July, of course, but I reasoned that it was better to wait until the New Year to start.

Every year I told myself that this was the year that I was going to change my life. Every year I was filled with hope.

Since I had so many bad habits to choose from—smoking, drinking, overeating, lack of exercise—I usually just picked the one I was most concerned about at the time. Some years I told myself I would stop smoking. Other years I resolved to lose weight. Once or twice I planned to get into shape.

Quitting smoking was easy. No problem. Although I had been a smoker most of my adult life, I still wasn't willing to accept that it was anything more than a bad habit. Addicted? Not me! After all, I had quit twenty or thirty times.

Losing weight was easy, too. I just stopped eating. Or at the very least I stopped eating all the foods I liked to eat and replaced them with foods I couldn't stand putting into my mouth.

I liked losing weight and I got very good at it. Unfortunately, I got even better at putting it back on. When you are carrying sixty, seventy, or eighty pounds more than your ideal weight, you've got plenty to work with. The beauty is, with that many extra pounds, almost any diet works . . . for a little while.

Losing weight satisfied the martyr in me. During the first few weeks of January, I would allow myself to feel a strange combination of self-pity and self-righteousness. I stood in judgment over those who didn't have the self-control that I had. Like any good martyr, I wore the wounds of self-denial as badges of courage.

I wasn't sure exactly what getting in shape meant, but I was pretty sure it had something to do with having a flat stomach, since everyone I saw who looked fit seemed to have a flat stomach. So all of my getting-in-shape programs began with doing sit-ups.

Once, in my early thirties, I actually tried to become a runner. I had an old friend who had become a marathoner and appeared to be a fairly normal person. He lost weight, looked great, and seemed more content than I had ever known him to be. I figured if he could run marathons, so could I. At the time, I had no idea that there was any other distance for a road race. If you were a runner, I thought, you ran marathons.

For a few painful months I tried to be a marathoner. I didn't read any books or magazines about running before I started. How complicated could running be? I reasoned. How much could there be to know? You just put one foot in front of the other, right?

Of course, none of my "get fit" plans lasted more than a few weeks. They never lasted until the spring thaw. In the course of my lifetime I became very accomplished at one thing though: I became very good at quitting.

A LIFE OF SEDENTARY CONFINEMENT

*F*inally I decided to stop resolving. I was getting older. As a friend of mine said, one day you wake up and realize that you have your father's (or mother's) body. But rather than working on changing, I worked on accepting the changes.

I looked for activities that required no movement. I sat at my desk and worked hard to buy things . . . things to sit on! I decided that leisure meant inactivity. I took great pride in my ability to avoid physical effort.

It's important to remember that for most of my life I was an expert at non-running. On my first day as a runner, I owned nine motorcycles, two cars, a camper, a garden tractor, a riding lawn mower, and a gas-powered weed-whacker.

I was never in danger of having to exert myself. I worked hard so I would not have to work hard. Breaking a sweat was something *other* people did—when they were working for me.

You may have fallen into the same trap I did. You may believe that physical activity is the province of the young and fit, that the deterioration of your body is the inescapable reality of living.

Who can blame us? Except for the rare fifteen second's achievement of some extraordinary senior citizen, often we never see anyone our age engaged in any form of physical activity. Instead, we see retirees enjoying their golden years in peaceful settings with their every need anticipated and satisfied.

In time, the athletes on television and in print become closer to our children's ages than to ours. We accept it as inevitable. We see athletes who are "old" at thirty and believe that our careers are over before they ever begin.

For me, with each passing year I got farther from being either young or fit. Suddenly it was five, then ten, then twenty years from that time when I thought I was in my prime. Without warning, I was old and overweight and out of shape. And I couldn't imagine life being any different.

My ever-widening waist and sagging arms were testimony to my accomplishments. I was a fat cat. I carried proudly the accumulated excesses of food and drink.

The obvious aging of my body was matched by the invisible aging of my soul. You can't see it and you can't feel it, but over time the soul becomes just as unwilling to work as the body does. As soft as I was getting on the outside, I was getting equally hard on the inside.

Although I didn't know it then, I was sad almost all of the time. I'm not talking about clinical depression or an emotional or psychological condition that would have responded to therapy. I was simply, completely, and essentially . . . sad. I had accepted that I could no longer expect to be happy, only content. I was tired, inside and out.

Now I see people who are sad and I want to tell them that it doesn't have to be that way. I see people who are carrying the physical and emotional weight of years of excess and I want to explain that the happiness they are so desperate for is only a few steps away.

They say you can't run away from your troubles. I say that you can.

MY MOMENT OF TRUTH

People ask if there was a particular moment of enlightenment that caused me to change. They are surprised to learn that there was no moment of epiphany, no blinding light. There was only the relentless march toward middle age.

There was one incident, though, that maybe would pass for an epiphany. I had been invited to a fancy dinner party and needed to rent a tuxedo. The salesperson measured my out seam. Forty inches. Then she measured my waist. Also forty inches!

I had become a cube! I had the measurements of a decent-sized throw rug.

And so, at age forty-three, when I found myself standing in my garage in a pair of new running shoes, I knew that it was my moment of truth. Surrounded by the mechanical witnesses to my folly, I stared out at my driveway and into my future. Ahead of me lay forty yards of driveway. Behind me lay forty years of bad decisions and broken promises.

I'm not sure how long I stood there. I was paralyzed by fear and more frightened of starting than I was of not starting. I knew that this was it. I knew that this would be the last time I would have the courage to start.

With a primal scream I started down the driveway, at a full sprint. Arms flailing and legs pumping, I ran like a person possessed. I guess I was. I ran at full speed toward tomorrow. For about thirty seconds!

That's as long as it took for my legs to hurt, my lungs to hurt, and my ego to hurt. I stopped dead in my tracks. Thirty seconds! That was as long as I could run. I was overcome with my own arrogance, and I started to laugh. After years of working hard and playing hard and living hard, I couldn't move my body for longer than thirty seconds.

It never occurred to me that I would stick with it. Why should this time be any different from the others? But I found myself putting on my running shoes, heading out the door, and waiting for the urge to quit to overcome me. As the days passed, and then weeks and months, I became perplexed. Surely I would quit. I always had in the past.

This time, though, something was different. Even now I'm not sure what made the difference. Running—well, okay, waddling— was becoming a part of my life. And I was enjoying it.

It may just have been the absurdity of it that kept me interested—the complete incongruity of "John the Runner" living in the body of "John the Couch Potato."

BECOMING A RUNNER

Whatever the reason, I continued to run. That is not to say that I considered myself a runner. No, I thought of myself only as a person who ran. After all, runners looked different from me. They were lean and fluid. I was thick and clumsy.

That I continued astounded me. Over the first days and weeks I shifted from walking for a while to mixing some running with the walking to mixing some walking with the running. I kept repeating that cycle until I kept myself moving for about thirty minutes at a time.

Still convinced that I would quit, I began to set goals for myself. When I could easily run a quarter of a mile, I tried for a half-mile. Much to my surprise, my body continued to adapt. Soon I was running a mile, then two, and finally three miles at a time, three days a week.

It wasn't pretty, but it was a start. I learned a lot in those first weeks. I learned that for me, like so many others, running is the answer. Out on the road it is just you, the pavement, and your will. Running is elementary. It is elegant in its simplicity.

As the effects of being a runner became more obvious, as I lost thirty, fifty, and eventually one hundred pounds, I wanted more. I wanted to race.

So I ran a 5K (3.1 miles), then a 10K (6.2 miles). As I accomplished these goals, I was forced to set new ones. I finished a half-marathon (13.1 miles), and eventually, much to my amazement, I finished a full marathon—26.2 miles! Still no sign of quitting. What had happened to me?

Make no mistake, I was still very slow. I was often last or nearly last. I was always the slowest in my age group. But I was there at the beginning and at the end of every race. As I crossed finish line after finish line, as the race numbers began to clutter my refrigerator door, and as my running shoes began to multiply like rabbits, I was forced to face the truth. I had become a runner. Now what? I had no plan for succeeding and almost no experience with self-congratulations and celebrations.

TELLING MY STORY

I began to tell my story on the Internet. The anonymity of sitting alone at my laptop protected me from my fear of being ridiculed. I started posting to a running discussion group. Slowly, I worked up the nerve to describe not only what I was doing but what I was feeling.

My first venture into writing was actually nothing more than an e-mail message. I told about a race, about finishing nearly last, and about what it felt like to be middle-aged, slow, but happy. It was the first time I had ever invited anyone to share the joy of my running.

Much to my surprise, several unseen friends e-mailed me back to say that I had told their stories, as well as my own. They told me that I had managed to put into words what they were feeling about themselves, about the metamorphosis in their lives, and about the role running played in their self-discovery.

Encouraged by their responses, I began sending an e-mail to the group every month. I called it "The Penguin Chronicles." The character of the penguin came from my own observation of my running style. I knew I wasn't a rabbit, but I didn't feel like a turtle, either. I needed a new image to capture the awkward but tenacious steps I was taking. Penguins, as they have come to be called, are runners of all shapes, sizes, ages, and genders. Some are fast. Most are not. But what unifies us as runners is out commitment to using running as a way to find the best in ourselves and those around us.

As I continued to tell my story, I discovered that I was not alone. I discovered that nearly everyone in the middle of the back of the pack at races is astounded to be there.

In the summer of 1997, I took yet another step. I strapped my running shoes to the back of my motorcycle and headed out to find myself and my friends. For nearly two months I ran alone and with groups, as slowly as I wanted and as fast as I could. I met Penguins from North Carolina to California and from Oregon to Washington, D.C.

In the summer of 1998, I hit the road again. This time I was in a car and I would be away from home for twelve weeks and cover 14,000 miles. I ran in the heat of Houston and in the morning chill of Squaw Valley. I ate in places with names like Bubba's and Whitey's. Every run in every new place was like a homecoming. My life would never be the same.

For many runners, it is as though we have been plucked from our previous lives and transported to a parallel universe—a Never-Never-Land where we are all Peter Pan. We are living lives that only a short time ago would have been a fantasy.

FINDING YOURSELF

I've given up on having a plan to succeed. With each step, with every mile, I am making a new plan. I may not be ready to accept success, but I am no longer prepared to quit. And I'll gladly accept the effort of being a runner. I'll challenge myself to run farther and to run faster. Because I know that the only person I will ever have to outrun is the person I used to be.

More than that, I have learned just how far I was from who I wanted to be. And from the day of that realization, every step has taken me closer to the person I am trying to become.

Starting is scary. It is for everyone. Joan Benoit-Samuelson, the U.S. women's marathon record holder, talks about how, as a new runner, she would stop running to pick flowers as cars passed by her because she was so embarrassed by how she looked. I never allowed my eyes to meet those of other runners, because I was afraid of seeming like an impostor.

In time, though, those fears subside. In time, as you begin to realize that it is the quality of your effort that matters, failure becomes unthinkable. How can you fail to become yourself?

Every runner has had to take that first step. Each of us in our own way has had to find that courage. So can you.

This is not a book about how to be a better runner. If you've never run, it provides some helpful tips to get you started. If you've run for a while, it contains some bits of collected wisdom that may help you run farther or faster. If you are an experienced runner, it may help you rediscover the joy of your early running years.

This is, in large part, a book about *why* to run. Whether you are simply thinking about beginning to run, or have been running for a week or a lifetime, this book will help you think differently about the activity of running and about the sport of running. This book will show, through my own experience and the experience of hundreds of others, how you can find the joy in running that we do.

In the pages of this book you will see yourself in the stories of other runners. You will discover that what you are feeling is shared by men and women, young and old. And you will understand that what we have in common as runners is more important than what separates us as individuals.

The Courage to Start is about how to use running as a means to find yourself. The road and the trails and the treadmill can become the paths that lead from who you are today to who you want to become tomorrow.

This book is also, by default more than design, a journal of a journey. It is the story of one person's trip back from middle age. It is the outline of an odyssey of hope and disappointment, of moving forward and falling back, of life-altering revelation and profound stupidity. It is the story of the search for my self and the remarkable joy of discovering that who I really am is much better than who I once pretended to be.

More important, it is the story of the people I have met on my journey. It is about runners who have shared their joys with me, who have laughed with me and cried with me. It is a story about the hundreds of intersections of my life and other people's and of the truths those people told me and that I have tried faithfully to pass on.

As the songwriter Paul Simon put it, "There were incidents and accidents, and in each there have been moments of revelation." This is true not just for me but for all those who have been kind enough and courageous enough to join me in my search. More than being my story, it is their story. It is our story.

2

Getting Off on the Right Foot

One of the most attractive aspects of running is that it seems so simple. There's no expensive equipment to buy, no need to drag that equipment someplace far away to use it, no need to get together with a partner or a team. All you really need is a pair of shoes and a place to run.

Of course, as I was to discover, it isn't quite that simple. Running shoes are complex feats of engineering designed to protect, support, correct, and enhance the runner's natural biomechanics. Finding the right shoe for your foot is not always easy.

But by my early reasoning, running should be a very natural activity. Certainly our ancestors had a running instinct. Humans are a nomadic people. For centuries they moved from place to place using only their feet. It is hard to imagine any community of humans that would not have included runners. Surely I could run, too.

I had seen evidence of the running instinct in children. I had even experienced the joy of running as a child myself. As a child, there were times when I seemed to be possessed by the pure act of running. I was content just to run. I didn't need a destination. I didn't have to be running to or from anything. I just wanted to run.

We've all seen children who appear to derive such pleasure from the act of running that they can't, or won't, stop. When my son was young, he would break into spontaneous episodes of running. If there was no room to run straight, he would run in circles like a whirling dervish. He got the "willies" when he had to sit still for too long.

When I am asked why I chose to start running after forty years of sedentary confinement, I answer that running is in my genes. Somewhere in my genetic makeup is the DNA residue of great hunters, warriors, and messengers. When I dig deep enough into my soul, I am connected directly to those who ran for their lives.

I'm not convinced, though, that all of my running ancestors were gifted runners. Some of them must have been more like me. Unlike world-class runners who have strides that are long and powerful, *my* running stride is almost exactly the length of my foot. Clearly, I am not a descendant of the fastest and the strongest.

The image in my head may be one of an Olympian, but the reality is that I run like a Penguin.

I am living proof that there have been slow runners—Penguin runners—throughout history! I suspect that the members of my ancestral tribe would *not* have selected me to chase down dinner. If they had, we would have become vegetarians by default. Given my running ability, it is far more likely that I would have ended up as some other animal's dinner.

MY FIRST RUNNING SHOES

Soon after I began running, I decided that in order to feel like a runner I needed to buy my first real pair of running shoes. I hadn't looked at running shoes, much less been to a running-shoe store, in years.

The last time I had thought about buying anything other than dress shoes, they were called "gym" shoes. In those days you had only two choices in athletic shoes: Keds or PF Flyers. Both came in either high-tops or low-tops.

Keds were the shoes with the blue rectangle on the heel. PF Flyers had a black rectangle. In my school, the serious athletes all had PF Flyers. If you were a basketball player, they were high-tops. I, on the other hand, had Keds. And they were low-top Keds. Even in elementary school, I was in the back of the pack.

Those rubber-bottomed canvas shoes weighed about six pounds each and were designed to prevent unrestrained youngsters from making marks on the wood floor of the gymnasium. I'm convinced that was their only real purpose. Well, no, there was one other . . . they made a great screeching sound when you stopped real fast. Although I never learned to shoot a basketball and I never learned to jump high or run fast, I could make a mean screech!

But I needed running shoes, so I found myself standing in front of an athletic-shoe store in the mall looking through the window at about eight thousand pairs of shoes. There were shoes for running and shoes for walking. And shoes for tennis and soccer and squash and nearly every other sport. Mostly, though, there were shoes for basketball.

And the shoes all had names! I'm sure they must have been the names of people who were famous basketball players, but all that was lost on me. What I saw was a collection of brightly colored shoes that appeared to have been designed on and shipped in from another planet.

I almost quit right then. How was I going to decide among all of these shoes? I had no idea what I wanted and I had even less of an idea of what I needed. I didn't even know enough to know how much I didn't know. I wanted to get out of there as fast as I could. I wanted to go home, sink back into my sofa, and never think about running again.

But before I could escape, a very friendly salesperson cornered me. "May I help you?" he asked politely. Not wanting to appear to be a complete idiot, I told him that I was looking for a *new* pair of running shoes. My plan, if you could call it that, was to fool him into thinking that I was looking for a replacement pair of running shoes. I did not want to admit to him what I had barely admitted to myself—I was without a clue.

"Wonderful!" he exclaimed. Then my worst fears were realized. I could tell he knew I was bluffing. He knew I had no idea what I was talking about. He did his best to be helpful, but suddenly he began speaking a language I didn't understand.

"Do you overpronate?" he asked. "Or do you supinate? Are you a heel-striker or a forefoot-striker?" He continued to barrage me with questions. "Do you need medial support? Are you looking for a stability shoe? A motion-control shoe? A cushioned shoe? Do you need a training shoe or a racing flat?"

I couldn't have been more embarrassed if I had been standing there naked. I had entered a world in which I knew nothing. I was out of place and everyone knew it. At least this seventeen-year-old knew it! And it hurt.

I'm not sure how long I stood there as I tried to think of an answer that would make sense, but eventually I simply looked at him and said that all I knew was that I needed a *left* shoe and a *right* shoe. He graciously brought me a pair of shoes that he thought would work, and mercifully sent me on my way.

THE "RIGHT" SHOE FOR YOU

Whether you're a new runner or an experienced runner, buying the correct shoe is probably the most important decision you will make. What's more, it's a decision that you have to make over and over. A shoe that works for the first six months of your running life may not work as you improve, get faster, or start running longer distances.

The correct shoe will enhance your natural stride and will help prevent injuries. It will allow your foot to strike the ground, move through its running motion, and push off with ease and in perfect harmony with your hips and knees.

The wrong shoe can turn running into a torturous routine of pain and recovery. The wrong shoe will force your foot out while your knee goes in, which is almost exactly the point at which your hip goes out. The wrong shoe sets up a battleground in your body between your muscles and tendons and bones and joints and can end your running program in a matter of days.

The problem becomes even more complex because there is no single shoe that is right for every runner. The activity of running, or at least getting started as a runner, would be much easier if you could just drop by the shoe store and buy a generic pair of beginner's running shoes. But our feet, our bodies, and our budgets are all different.

There are, however, some general guidelines. These descriptions are not intended to be the definitive word on foot motion and shoe construction. They are intended to help you avoid that moment of embarrassment and the feeling of abject ignorance that I had with the young shoe salesman. They are intended to allow you to ask the right questions.

Pronation: This is the foot's natural tendency to roll inward as you run. The perfect foot begins the running or walking motion somewhat on the outside of the heel and rolls inward toward the ball of the foot.

Overpronation: This is what happens when the foot rolls inward too far. The beginning of the running motion often is fine, but the foot continues to roll inward too far, beyond the ball of the foot.

Supination: This refers to what happens when the foot does not roll inward enough. As you walk or run, the striding motion occurs entirely along the outside of the foot.

Oversupination: This is what happens when the foot rolls outward too much as it moves through the running motion.

What does all of this mean? What good is it to know these words if you don't know why you need to know them? How can you tell which labels apply to your feet and your running stride?

YOUR FOOT

You can make a preliminary judgment about your foot by looking at the shoes that you wear most often. Find a pair of your favorite shoes. They don't have to be running shoes. A pair of shoes that you have worn long enough for the wear pattern on the bottom of the shoes to be visible will do. Set the shoes on a flat surface so that you can inspect them from behind. Look carefully at the wear pattern, especially in the heel.

If all of your shoes are worn slightly on the outside of the heel and the inside of the sole, chances are that your foot pronates normally. If the heels of your shoes are worn badly on the inside but not on the outside, it's likely that you are an overpronator. If the outside of your heels and soles are worn, you are probably a supinator.

You can also take the wet-foot test if you want more information. With the bottoms of your feet wet (but not soaked), step onto a piece of paper. If the imprint of your foot looks like a foot, you probably pronate normally. If the imprint looks like one large blob, you probably have flat feet and may need motion-control shoes. If you see separate marks for your heel and the ball of your foot, with nothing connecting them, chances are you have high arches and may be able to run comfortably in stable or cushioned shoes.

Once you've determined what kind of foot you have, the next step is to buy a pair of shoes that are appropriate for your foot. It's not really all that complicated.

TYPES OF SHOES

Motion-control shoes do exactly what they say they do. These shoes are designed to prevent the foot from rolling inward. This is accomplished by using different materials or placing devices in the sole of the shoe. If you overpronate—that is, if your foot rolls inward too much—a motion-control shoe can help. These shoes tend to be rather stiff and generally don't have much cushioning. Runners with flat feet often do well in motion-control shoes.

Stability shoes have more cushioning than motion-control shoes but are still designed to prevent excessive pronation. These shoes usually provide support for the inner (medial) part of the foot. Runners with normal feet, or those who pronate just a little too much, do well in stability shoes.

Cushioned shoes feel the softest when you run. They may feel so wonderful that you think you are running on clouds, but they provide little or no support and don't control foot motion at all. These shoes work best for the biomechanically blessed runner who does not overpronate or oversupinate.

Unfortunately, the very softness of cushioned shoes can lead to problems. If the foot rolls inward or outward too much, a cushioned shoe won't do anything to prevent the excessive roll. Even though they feel great at first, shoes that are too soft can lead to pain in the knees as your joints struggle to keep the foot from rolling inward or outward.

Since so few runners supinate, or roll to the outside of the foot, there aren't nearly as many shoe choices for this type of foot. If you supinate, you will want to avoid shoes designed to prevent the foot from rolling in, because they will just make your problem worse. Look for shoes that enhance the foot's natural tendency to roll inward.

The importance of wearing shoes that fit properly cannot be overemphasized. Typically, your running shoes will be a half to a full size larger than your dress shoes. But there is very little consistency in sizing among brands of running shoes. You may wear a size nine in one model, an eight and a half in another, and a nine and a half in still another. The sizing is even less consistent between shoe manufacturers. Forget the size. Buy the shoe that fits.

A good rule of thumb is the rule of thumb. When you are standing, you should have a space the width of your thumb between the end of your longest toe and the end of your shoe. *Always* remember that it's much better to wear a running shoe that's a little too long than one that's a little too short. You can always buy thicker socks, which provide more cushion, if the shoe is a bit too long.

Modern running shoes are far superior to the gym shoes of my childhood. By using a little common sense, you can make your first, or next, shoe-buying experience much more pleasant. With a little practice, you'll find that you're able to use words like overpronation and medial support along with the experts.

Most cities have running specialty stores with qualified salespeople who will help you select the best shoe for your feet. Often these stores are owned and staffed by runners. Although you may be intimidated at first, they really are there to help you become a runner. If you find a store with staff who don't want to help a new runner, use your old shoes to walk to a different store!

THE WELL-DRESSED RUNNER

Almost every runner seems to start running in the same outfit— an old pair of sweatpants and an oversized T-shirt. If you're shaped like I was, it's even better if that T-shirt is long enough to cover your belly and your behind. I would have run in a rain poncho if I had thought it would cover more of me.

Eventually it becomes clear that being a runner means buying running clothes. *Real* running clothes—shirts and shorts that are designed to work with a body that is in motion and clothes that are made of materials that will make you more comfortable.

Experienced runners will tell you there are only two conditions in which we run: weather that is either too hot or too cold. In either case, it also may be too rainy, too windy, too dry, too humid, and so on. The conditions are rarely ideal.

High-quality running clothes are designed to close the gap between the real conditions and the ideal. They are designed to keep you cool, or warm, or dry. Different manufacturers have different names for fabrics, such as CoolMax, Polartec, Dryline, and Dri-F.I.T., that accomplish this. They all try to perform the same functions: to help the body control its temperature and to keep your body dry.

Regardless of the outside temperature, your body heats up with effort. In warm weather, a lightweight shirt made of something like CoolMax will help pull the sweat away from your body, allowing you to stay cool. In cold weather, that same material worn under a wind-blocking shell, will pull the moisture away from your body to the next layer of clothing to help keep you warm.

The same principle applies to every piece of clothing you wear when you run, including shorts, socks, and underwear. Look for words like "wicking," which simply means drawing moisture away from the skin.

In cold weather the secret is to layer lightweight garments so that the clothing works together to keep you dry and warm. Materials like polypropylene and polar fleece are designed to keep the body temperature steady, while wicking the moisture away from your skin to the surface layer of clothing. Because these fabrics wick rather than absorb moisture, your clothes don't get soggy and heavy as you sweat.

At first, your new running clothes may not seem as comfortable as that old pair of sweats and oversized T-shirt, but in time you'll get used to the lightness and breathability of these new clothes. And you may just find that you look REALLY good in neon green!

FINDING THE TIME

As important as having the right running shoes is, it is only the beginning. Getting your shoes is quite literally only the first step. What you do with those shoes and how you feel about yourself when you're wearing those shoes will ultimately determine whether you will continue to run.

Getting off on the right foot means understanding enough about yourself, your life, and your willingness to commit to this new activity to begin to think about your life as a runner. It's about giving yourself permission to find the time to be a runner.

Time is often a big factor, particularly in the early days and weeks of our running lives. Many of us are already so busy that it's hard to imagine adding another time-consuming activity to our overstuffed schedules, although running is one of the most time-efficient exercises around. You need to find a strategy that will allow you to make time for it.

If you are new to running or being active, one of the best ways to get started is to take an entire week to think about running. Each day that week, think about when and where you might have run that day. Think about how fast or how far you would run. Remind yourself that NEXT week, you really are going to run.

In the beginning, running doesn't need to take a lot of time. In the first few months, try to establish a schedule. You are more likely to succeed if you find just a few minutes several times a week that you can commit to running than if you devise an elaborate and completely undoable schedule that will fall apart in a matter of days.

Plan your runs on the basis of time rather than distance. Plan to get out of the house for a certain amount of time. Forget how far you go. Forget how fast you go. Just get out the door and stay out. For many people, twenty minutes of activity is a good place to begin. That does not mean running for twenty minutes. It means staying on your feet moving forward for twenty minutes. If you can run, run. If you can walk, walk. Do whatever you can, but keep moving forward. If it gets too hard, slow down.

A good beginning program would look like this:

Week One: On 3 non-consecutive days, get out of your house and move for 20 minutes.

Week Two: On 3 non-consecutive days, get out of your house and move for 25 minutes.

Week Three: On 3 non-consecutive days, get out of your house and move for 30 minutes.

Week Four: On 4 non-consecutive days, get out of your house and move for 20 minutes.

Week Five: On 4 non-consecutive days, get out of your house and move for 25 minutes.

Week Six: On 4 non-consecutive days, get out of your house and move for 30 minutes.

Week Seven: On 5 days, get out of your house and move for 20 minutes.

Week Eight: On 5 days, get out of your house and move for 25 minutes.

Week Nine: On 5 days, get out of your house and move for 30 minutes.

This program makes no prescriptions for mileage or speed. If you follow this program for nine weeks, regardless of how fast or how far you go, you will be well on your way to making movement a part of your life.

A program of alternating running and walking is also a good way to begin. The first week that may mean running for thirty seconds and walking for five minutes to recover. In time, it may mean running one minute and walking five, or running one and walking one. The truth is, it doesn't matter. What matters is that you are learning to use your body as a means of transportation.

Improvement is defined as being closer to where you want to be than you are right now. Remember, I couldn't run for more than a few steps in the beginning. Improvement for me was running farther than my driveway. You'll have to decide what improvement means for you. Is it to walk around your block without stopping? Then work toward that!

For better or worse, you are the only you that you will ever get. What you decide to do with you is up to you. Tomorrow you will still be you. The question is whether you will move closer today to who you want to be.

If you are patient, if you are persistent, if you are consistent, an amazing transformation will begin to occur. Your wonderfully adaptive body will begin to cooperate. It will happen in your own time and at your own pace, to be sure, but the transformation will take place.

Movement, which may have seemed so foreign to you, will become more natural. Being active every day will stop being something that you want to end and become something that you can't wait to start. It isn't just a matter of going farther or faster every day. It's knowing that you are in control of your body and, for a few minutes every day, your life.

You are becoming a runner. You are becoming a person for whom the activity of running is no longer completely foreign. Those brand-new running shoes will begin to show signs of wear. Those once bright white running socks will become dulled by the sweat of your transformation.

Not only are you becoming a runner, but you are becoming a runner in training. You will have goals. You will have good days and bad days. You will have days when you can't wait to run and days when you will have to force yourself out the door. In other words, you will be just like all the other runners. Every day you will be trying to do your best.

MEASURES OF EFFORT

What is most often misunderstood about those of us who are struggling to reach the front of the back of the pack is that we really are trying. We really are, at whatever our pace, doing the best we can. Some runners, and even some well-meaning non-runners, interpret our position in the back of the pack as a measure of our lack of effort. Nothing could be further from the truth.

We—the few, the proud, the plodding—very often train as much or more than faster runners. At a blistering twelve- (or even ten-) minute pace, a fifteen mile week represents a major time commitment. In order to prepare for a race, I do speed work and tempo runs and I do long slow runs. I just do them very slowly!

It's not a matter of trying harder. And it's not a matter of training longer. It's not a matter of lack of motivation, either. It's just a matter of speed. A friend of mine—a fast runner—put it succinctly when I asked him what he thought the limiting factor in my running future was. His answer was as insightful as it was concise. "Maybe you're just slow!"

Slow I may be. If you are new to running, you may be, too. But by accepting the challenges presented to you by your choices and your genetics, you can work at becoming the best runner you know how to be. Every day gives you an opportunity to improve. With every run, you can try to be better. Not just a better runner, but a better person.

Now is the time to give in to your running instinct. Today is the day to let go of all the unrealistic expectations and uncover the primal joy in running. It may be that, like me, the more you run, the more connected you will feel to your running ancestors.

Before you know it, there will be times when you will imagine yourself running free across the plains or silently through the forest. You'll be able to imagine yourself being chosen to deliver the news of some important victory to a distant people. You will see yourself running strong and well.

As true as it is that the journey of a thousand miles begins with a single step, so, too, does the journey to a new life as a runner. Every day that you run, you are one step closer to wherever you're headed.

3

Body of Evidence

I don't have a runner's body. Or at least I didn't think I did at first. My image of a runner's body was one with long spindly legs, narrow hips, pencil-thin arms, and with skin that looked like it was attached directly to the skeleton.

It wasn't that I knew many runners, or even that I had seen that many. It was, I suppose, mostly a matter of what I imagined runners looked like. In my imagination they looked very different from me.

You may be clinging to that image of a runner's body as I did—as an excuse for not becoming a runner. It's the perfect deception. When the thought of running crosses your mind, you simply try to imagine yourself as a runner. You picture your body in running shorts. You picture yourself exposing that much skin to people you don't know. That's usually enough to end the dream.

I asked myself how I could be expected to run with my short, stubby little legs. How could anyone who had spent his entire life buying pants designed with a "little" more room in the seat and thighs be a runner? How could a person whose waist and inseam were almost the same be a runner?

I told myself that people who were "big-boned" could never be runners, so there was no sense in trying. Sure, I might lose weight. I might even get fitter. But no matter how good the shape I was in, I convinced myself that I would never be the "shape" of a runner.

Your body may seem peculiar to you, too. It may be that you

think your legs are the problem, as I did. Or it might be your thighs, or hips, or your belly that don't fit the image. You look at your unique combination of body parts and are convinced that they can never be made to run. You are probably wrong!

I can say that because I was wrong. I was wrong in thinking that runners had a particular kind of body and wrong in thinking that my body could not become the body of a runner. I was wrong in limiting what I could be by imagining only what I thought I could *not* be.

Your shape could be the shape of a runner. Your body, for all of its shortcomings and excesses, could still be the body of a runner. After all, if you run with your body . . . it becomes the body of a runner.

Runners come in every imaginable shape and size. I have been passed in races by tall runners and short runners. I have been passed by runners who look as though they have not eaten in six weeks, and by runners who appear to have just wiped out an all-you-can-eat breakfast bar.

Standing at the starting line of my first race I couldn't believe my eyes. At first glance, it was hard to tell who was running and who was there to cheer on the runners. There were men and women, young and old, short and tall gathered to test their bodies and spirits. And some of them were *not* so thin.

IMAGES OF FITNESS AND HEALTH

Much of my confusion about what a runner's body looked like—in fact, most of my confusion about what a fit body looked like—came from the images of health and fitness portrayed in the media. Those images, and the constantly changing definitions of fitness and health, led me to believe that it was hopeless for me to think about becoming either fit or healthy.

I didn't realize that our bodies are wonderfully adaptive. Almost as soon as we begin to alter our level of activity, our bodies begin to change. If we continue to require greater strength or greater endurance from our bodies, our bodies will adapt. Whether we accept it or not, the bodies we have are the products of what we have required them to be.

For the better part of forty years I had spent nearly all day every day sitting. In time, my body got very good at sitting. I sat at my job, I sat riding to and from my job, and I sat when I got home. If I went anywhere, I sat when I got there.

You may be taking great pride, as I did, in not having to do anything. You may be working extra hours to buy the kinds of things that will allow you to do less and less. You may be convinced that the real goal of working hard is to get to the point where you don't have to do a thing.

Unfortunately, in time, we become prisoners in our own bodies. We become prisoners not so much because of the way our bodies look, although that, too, is a problem. We are prisoners in bodies that are becoming less and less able to do anything.

In my case, after forty years of sedentary confinement I no longer was able to enjoy the activities that I had enjoyed in the past. There were things that I once was able to do that I simply couldn't do anymore.

When I did use my body—to till the garden or clean the garage—I often was sore for days afterward. When I resisted the temptation to do nothing and pressed my body into service, I paid for it dearly with fatigue and lingering pain. With each episode of aching, I told myself that I would never do anything to provoke that pain again.

Like many others, I believed that the single most important measurement of my body was my weight. I believed the expression "You can never be too thin or too rich." I looked enviously at those around me who weighed less and, consequently, were valued more in our world.

Many new runners want to know how many calories are burned

by running. They want to calculate the amount of effort used and the amount of weight that they can lose. They believe that being thinner guarantees being happier, healthier, and fitter.

It doesn't. There is no direct correlation between being thin and being healthy or fit. If being healthy is defined as the absence of disease, then it's clear that a thin body isn't always a healthy body. By the same token, if being fit is a function of how efficiently the body uses oxygen and transports blood, then being heavy is not the same as being unfit.

The standard by which we measure ourselves and our fitness cannot be based exclusively on weight. Because we are runners, it is what our bodies can do that is important—not what those bodies look like.

THE "SHAPE" OF OUR BODIES

My body, like yours, is the aggregate of hundreds of years of genetic experimentation, of men and women who found each other attractive and combined their gene pools to produce new generations. Over time, the possible genetic combinations reach staggering proportions. The result for you and me is a body that includes reminders of hundreds of our ancestors.

When eventually I looked objectively at my body, when I looked past what I wanted it to be and took a more sympathetic and historical view, I understood that I am the product of a combination of many, diverse body types.

My legs must have come from a people who were less than three feet high, while my trunk and arms came from folks well over six feet five inches tall. My legs, trunk, and arms don't really go together well. It's as though my body were assembled from leftover parts.

It was only as I began to run and to meet other runners that I saw that the shape of our bodies is their least important feature. If you are pear-shaped, which many of us are, you have to become a lean and fit pear. If you are a beanpole, then be a strong beanpole.

What I didn't understand, and what many new runners don't understand, is that the most important parts of my body were the parts I couldn't see. While I spent all of my time looking at my too-short legs and too-long arms, it was the body inside the body that was taking shape.

It was the muscles and tendons and blood vessels that eventually changed my body once and for all. It was the stronger heart and tighter muscles that made my body what it needed to be. In time, I began to understand that it is the me inside of me that is the most important.

Your unique combination of heart and lungs and arms and legs is the same basic structure as every great athlete's. When you see people who appear to be stronger, or fitter, or healthier looking, don't be fooled into thinking that their bodies are structured any differently than yours. They may look different. Their random assortment of body parts may be arranged differently than yours, but they are not different.

Think about the greatest physical achievement you have ever witnessed or even heard of. Maybe it was climbing Mount Everest, or completing a marathon. Think about the person who accomplished that feat. How was that person different from you? How was he or she the same?

It may surprise you to know that no human physical achievement, no matter how extraordinary, was accomplished by someone with a body that was fundamentally different from yours and mine. All of the extraordinary feats of courage or tenacity or will were done by people just like you. That same potential resides in your body. It's just a matter of tapping into it.

It's easy to excuse yourself from dreaming of physical accomplishments if you believe that your body can't be different than it is. But it can. It can be stronger, firmer, and more powerful. And when it is, you'll begin to consider all of the possibilities. Where you once saw only the differences between bodies, you will soon celebrate their sameness.

RUNNING WITH THE BODY YOU HAVE

*E*verything changed the day I understood that if I was to become a runner, I would have to run with the body I had. The day I started to accept that my running goals would have to be accomplished with my feet attached to my legs, breathing air with my lungs, and pumping blood with my heart, every aspect of my running became more pleasurable and more satisfying.

This may sound obvious. Maybe it is to those who are much smarter or much less stubborn than I. But the truth is that, from the beginning, I believed that by dieting and exercising, in whatever form, I would get a different body. I believed that sometime in the middle of the night my old body would be replaced by a new one.

I would feel sillier about believing that I was going to get a different body if I didn't think that so many other people share my delusion. There is an industry devoted to promoting this illusion. There are machines and devices that are designed to convince you that you can have someone else's legs, or arms, or abdominal muscles.

There are television shows and infomercials that take advantage of our insecurities with our bodies. They go to great lengths to convince us that if we will do something for five minutes a day, three times a week, we will actually have someone else's body. I may have been silly, but I was not alone.

Eventually, I began to look at my body less as an object and more as a tool. I began to ask myself not what I wanted my body to look like, but what I wanted my body to be able to do. I stopped looking so much at the shape of particular parts of my body and instead started considering their function. I discovered that, indeed, my body was a well-designed, fully functioning machine.

My legs were neither too short nor too long. They were fine. They were attached to my hips. They had knees, which allowed them to bend. And my feet seemed to fit rather nicely on the ends of my legs.

Not only did my legs work, but, as it turned out, the rest of my body worked well, too. My lungs drew in air. My heart pumped blood. Every system in my body worked in concert with the others. I just needed to give my body a chance to function like a machine.

As I began to use my body, as it began to respond to the physical demands I was placing on it, I saw that change and improvement were a never-ending process. I finally understood that getting in shape wasn't something that you *did*. It was something that you are *always* doing.

I watched in amazement as my body began to refine itself into the product of my effort. I was stunned when I realized that it was my body that was bringing so much pleasure into my life. Rather than being my enemy, my body was trying to reestablish the friendship that I had long ago abandoned. Rather than sending me messages of despair, through fatigue and pain, my body was sending me messages of hope and exhilaration. My body was reasserting itself. My body was taking control.

FOOD AS FUEL

Almost without warning I began to think of food as fuel for my body, and not comfort for my soul. Food wasn't a new diet or a new program to lose weight. Food was part of the overall metamorphosis of my body from vessel to vehicle. As I wanted to do more with my body, I wanted to provide the fuel my body demanded.

The body has three sources of fuel: carbohydrates, protein, and fat. Carbs, as they are called, are the fast-acting, fast-burning fuel. Your body uses carbs quickly; consequently they need to be replaced often. Your body cannot store vast amounts of carbohydrates, so they are used or converted into a form that can be stored. Sources of carbohydrates include breads and cereals, fruits and vegetables, and anything else that seems "starchy."

Proteins burn more slowly than carbohydrates, but more quickly than fats. Sources for protein include meats, nuts, beans, and dairy products. Protein is found on the body as muscle.

Fat is everything that isn't protein or carbohydrate. Fat is exactly what it is called: FAT. If it looks like fat and feels like fat, it IS fat. The good news is that the body is very good at storing fat. We would never have survived harsh winters or food shortages if we weren't good at storing fat. The bad news is that our bodies are good at storing fat even if there is no shortage of food.

The body's number-one job is to keep you alive. Our bodies trust us. If you put too much food into your body, it believes that it's getting more food because you KNOW that there is going to be a food shortage. So your body starts stockpiling food. Your body stores the excess food as fat.

If you create an artificial food shortage, by going on an extreme diet or reducing your food intake below a healthy threshold, your wonderful body keeps you alive by slowing down your metabolism and using the reserves VERY slowly.

The key is to work with your body. You've got to provide the right balance of carbohydrates, proteins, and fats, combined with activity, that your body needs. Many dietary guidelines and exercise programs have features that may work for some of us, but not all of us. Trust yourself. Trust your body. Find your own balance.

In time you'll also understand that what you put into your body has a direct and immediate effect on how your body feels and performs. The food that you use as recreation or comfort is actually being used by your body as fuel. No less than any machine, your body requires the proper fuel in the proper balance. It couldn't be more simple.

If you always feel sluggish after eating certain foods, those foods are NOT the ideal choice for fuel before running or racing. If you are always hungry during your runs, you may need to eat more before you run or find foods that you can eat during a run. The time to diet, if you insist on using that word, is NOT during your runs.

As I began to consider the effect of food on my body, I began to see how a momentary indiscretion with food or drink could require enormous effort on the part of my body. I understood that my body would have to pay the consequences for my indiscretions. I understood that my body would function better if I was smarter about what I put into it.

If I overate or ate too much of what my body didn't need, I had to give it time and energy to process that food. That was wasted time. My body had to spend too much time processing food, and not enough time using the food as fuel. Without ever thinking DIET, I stopped overeating.

Transforming a body that has become accustomed to inactivity into one that willingly, even eagerly, runs does not happen overnight. At first, your body rebels. It sends messages, by way of aches and pains, that it is not pleased with the new program. It resists the change. It gets tired quickly and it waits impatiently for you to give up.

Before long, though, your body begins to get the message and it begins to adapt to the new stresses being placed on it. It does so by getting stronger. By carefully alternating between stress and recovery, your body actually becomes both more and less than it was.

As I've continued to run, as I've gotten to see and know more runners, I have learned that there is no such thing as a runner's body. There are only bodies that run. Mine, stubby legs and all, is the body of runner. Yours is, too. And it will become the body of a runner as you continue to use it to run.

4

Great Expectations

As I meet more runners and hear their stories, I'm convinced that the number-one reason people fail to stay with a running program is not lack of talent or discipline or time. What most often leads to failure is unrealistic expectations.

It's almost never a lack of talent. If all you are interested in doing, initially, as is true for most folks, is running or walking for the physical and mental health benefits, it doesn't take much talent. It's just a matter of getting out there and putting one foot in front of the other.

It's not a lack of discipline. Many new runners I speak with are highly successful professional people, or parents who have raised families, or folks who have achieved some measure of success and recognition in other areas. They have shown that they have the discipline to stay with a task and to see it through to its completion.

It's not a matter of being unable to find the time. Again, people who choose to begin a running program are often those for whom time management has become almost second nature. Many of them are already juggling multiple lives as husbands and wives, fathers and mothers, cooks and chauffeurs, while holding down a full-time job.

It's not any of these things. What causes so many well-intentioned new runners to abandon their new activity is unrealistic expectations. They decide, or are told, that they should be working toward objective mileage goals. They decide, or are told, that they should be aspiring to specific speed goals. Before long, the activity that started as a joyous adventure into a life of fitness has become just one more source of stress in an already over-stressed life.

It rarely starts that way. In the first days and weeks of running, most of us are so amazed that we are actually doing something physical that we aren't inclined to think about anything else. We are pleased that we have made a positive decision about our health and fitness. We are happy for having chosen to invest in our selves.

We also are so amazed that our bodies are adjusting and adapting to the new stresses that we have placed on them that we are in an almost constant state of delight. In the first few weeks of running, the improvements are dramatic. Each time we run we are discovering new challenges to overcome.

MOVING IN THE RIGHT DIRECTION

The truth is that starting a running program is easy. And because starting a running program doesn't require special skills or talent, running is often the last resort for those who have started and quit other sports and fitness programs. Because all you need is a pair of shoes and a place to run, people are often drawn to running after they discover the inconveniences of other forms of aerobic activity.

Running—unlike sports that require a partner, or expensive equipment, or learning a new set of skills, or traveling to where the activity can be practiced—is easy to integrate into one's life. It's quick, it's convenient, and it's simple.

Running doesn't have to become just another entry in a long list of false starts. With a little care and a little common sense, running can become the one activity that starts as fun and stays that way.

It's important to have goals. We all like to have goals. We like to know that if we get to this point by that time, we are on track. Setting goals is fun, but setting rigid goals can be disastrous.

Moving in the right direction, however slow your progress may be, is more important than setting arbitrary goals. If you examine the last week or month or year of your life and discover that you've been headed in the direction of more activity and better eating, then you can be certain you are getting closer to your fitness goal.

In the long run, it doesn't matter if it takes thirty or fifty weeks to reach that goal as long as you are going in the right direction. You haven't failed if you don't reach the magic weight or run the magic number of miles this week. Adjust your expectations, keep taking one step at a time, and you'll get there!

SOMETIMES IT'S HARD!

The litany of the emotional benefits of running is well known. Many of us like to philosophize about the inner peace produced by running. We like to tell ourselves and others how we use running as a means to self-discovery and enlightenment, how running reveals the truths about ourselves and the universe, and how through running we achieve cosmic unity. All of that may be true, but the physical and emotional benefits are only half the truth.

The other half is that sometimes running is difficult. Yes, you heard it here first. Sometimes running can feel like the most awkward activity anyone ever invented. Sometimes getting two feet and two legs pointed in the same direction is painful.

It's also true that not every run is fun. Blasphemy? Perhaps. But if you ask veteran runners to be completely honest, all of them will tell you the truth: sometimes you just want it to be over. There's no enlightenment, no cosmic connectedness. No nothing.

New runners seldom grasp the whole truth—that some days even those committed to running choose not to run. I can't explain it, but it happens. As much as running has brought to my life, there are days when I just can't make myself run. So I don't.

Why don't I run? Most often it's because there is nothing good that can come from running that day. I don't want to hate running. I don't want to force myself to run. There are too many things in my life that I *have* to do. Running will never be one of them—it is my choice.

In time, you will be able to distinguish between the days when you don't feel like running but should and the days when you do feel like running and shouldn't. In time, true wisdom will overcome you on those days when you feel like running . . . and know that you shouldn't. That's the first step to running for the rest of your life.

Understanding the whole truth is not easy for new runners. It wasn't easy for me either. I had no more idea of how to start than you may have. What I know now and what I want you to know is that if you are patient, the truth about what's best for you—in your life and in your running—will become clear. If you're like me, you will learn most of those lessons slowly.

I've met some new runners who don't want, or choose not, to believe the whole truth. It's easier for them to believe that they will magically reach new physical and emotional goals through running than to believe that reaching those goals will require patience, discipline, and plain hard work.

I've also met many experienced runners who don't want, or choose not, to believe the whole truth. They are the runners who are taped together, who are braced and elastic-bandaged from toe to waist. So, it is not just new runners who fail to listen to their bodies. My hope is that by getting rid of your unrealistic expectations you'll be less likely to do more when less would be better.

THE ROAD TO DISCOURAGEMENT

*F*or the most part, moving our bodies feels good. Even with a few aches and pains, even with the strange sensations that overtake our bodies, even with the sounds of our lungs struggling to get in enough air—it still feels good. We know that this is the right thing to be doing.

Unfortunately, the joy doesn't always last. All too soon the thrill of our own success is replaced by our need to compare ourselves to others. No longer satisfied with the miracle that is occurring in our lives, we begin to look at our relative place and pace in the running world. Our best is no longer good enough.

This shouldn't come as a surprise. We are told from childhood to do our best, but we know that *our* best is rarely good enough. We learned quickly that there was always a goal just beyond our reach that someone else had accomplished already, that we could reach if we *really* did our best. When our best fell short, as it often did, we were consoled by "Well, at least you tried."

We should remember that before children are taught that it is possible for them to be better or worse than someone else, they generally are quite content with their abilities. They accept, without complaint, the frustration of trying to learn to talk, crawl, walk, and use the bathroom. A young child is completely unaware that he/she is two weeks behind the normal developmental schedule. Children know only that the process is occurring at a pace that is suited to their needs and desires.

The road to discouragement begins with a single word: SHOULD. As soon as the word "should" appears in our thinking about our running, we are in trouble. When we think we "should" be able to run faster, or that we "should" be able to run farther, we have often taken the first step on the path to frustration and failure.

Sometimes it begins when a well-meaning friend, often a seasoned runner, begins to outline a training program and introduces the new runner to the word "should." Armed with the accumulated wisdom and expectations of a hundred running books and training guides, this friend explains just how far and how fast the new runner "should" be running every day.

When people ask me how far or how fast they "should" run, I ask them how far and how fast they "can" run. The secret to being successful at a running program is to take how far and how fast you "can" run, ask yourself how far and how fast you *want* to run, and then learn to live with narrowing the gap between what you "can" do and what you "want" to do.

Ask yourself how far you can run today. Be honest. It may be a quarter of a mile, it may be a marathon. Whatever it is, that's where YOU are as a runner. It doesn't make you a better or worse runner. It just tells you where you are as a runner.

All of us are somewhere. Like a good friend used to say "Wherever you are, there you are." If you don't like where you are, it's better to accept where you are and decide to move toward where you want to be than to berate yourself for where you are. I know very few runners, either recreational or professional, who will tell you that they are happy with where they are. Even if today is your first day as a runner, you share one quality with runners everywhere. You want to be better.

By starting with where you are and deciding on where you want to be, you can avoid the pitfalls of the "should's." You can avoid, from the very beginning, giving yourself feedback that is either falsely positive because you can exceed the "should's" or falsely negative because you can't meet the "should" standards. The alternative to accepting where you are and seeking only to improve is that you set yourself up for failure.

SETTING THE STAGE FOR FAILURE

How can I say this with such conviction? Because setting the stage for failure is exactly what I did. By setting my expectations so high that they were unachievable, I guaranteed I wouldn't meet them. By telling myself that in just a few weeks I could undo the damage I'd done to my body for forty-three years, I guaranteed I'd be disappointed.

I also began to set unrealistic time goals. In the first weeks, it was enough to finish a mile, and later, to complete a 5K race. But I expected my times to improve dramatically. Instead of being satisfied with a thirty-minute 5K, I was discouraged by my time and finishing position. I wanted to be better.

For too many new runners, this is the pattern. And for many it leads to frustration and, ultimately, to giving up. Had they waited the extra week or month or year it sometimes takes, these new runners probably would have found the joy they were looking for in their running.

There's no way to predict when the moment of enlightenment will occur. New runners have told me that they knew from the very first run that they would be runners for life. Other runners have told me that they have been running for a long time and still don't like it, in fact hate every step.

I can't tell you when that moment will come, but I can assure you that it's out there somewhere. A moment will come when you will forget that you are running and notice the sunrise or a flower. Another runner will approach and acknowledge *you* as a runner. A conversation will occur in which someone in your life refers to you as a runner. In that instant, running will change from an activity to a lifestyle.

Over the course of my lifetime I became very good at establishing unrealistic goals. Most of us have gotten caught in this trap. We tell ourselves that we will make a certain amount of money by a certain age or live in a certain size house or own a certain kind of car. (By the time I was thirty, I wanted to have a new Cadillac. At fifty, I still don't have it.) Expectations like these are just watersheds for failure.

It isn't only new runners who choose never to be satisfied with what they can achieve. Runners at the elite levels are also prone to view every run or race as an opportunity to berate their performance and themselves. Many of them seem to feel that if they accept honestly who they are, they will suddenly cease to be.

GOOD DAYS AND BAD DAYS

Only after I had injured myself time after time by trying to do what I told myself I "should" be able to do did the truth begin to sink in. For me, it took limping around on sore knees and achy legs. It took having to take days and weeks off from running in order to heal before I started to see the light.

Only after I began asking myself what I was capable of on that particular day or week did I begin to make any real progress. When I finally accepted who I was, I began to become who I wanted to be. When I finally gave myself permission to fail, I started to succeed.

As I got ready to run I would inventory my body and my soul. I would go through a physical and emotional checklist. It was a pre-flight inspection of both my ability and my willingness to run on that particular day.

By being honest with myself, I discovered that I wasn't the same person every day and that I wasn't the same runner every day. There were days when my body was eager to run, but my mind was so distracted by life that I found it difficult to enjoy the run. On other days, my soul desperately needed to run away but my body simply didn't have another mile in it.

I also discovered that my development and improvement as a runner were not linear. I didn't get a little better every day, the way I thought I would. My improvements came in fits and spurts. On some days easy was hard, and on others hard was easy. Often, it seemed that the improvements I thought I had made had evaporated by the next day.

One of the telltale signs of new runners is that they focus on getting faster on a certain route that they run. Don't worry; I did it, too. At first it took me forty minutes, then thirty-five, then thirty. I was improving and I knew it. Nearly every run was a PR (personal record) because I had so much room to improve.

Once you've overcome the momentum of your own inactivity, the improvements are much more incremental and there are ups and downs. You begin to have good days and bad days. In time you come to accept these fluctuations as natural.

As I began to be realistic with my expectations for myself as a runner, I was more realistic with myself as a person. I learned that my growth as a person wasn't any more linear than my improvement as a runner. In my spirit, as well as my body, there were days when I was much better than the day before and there were days when I had very little to offer.

By letting go of the expectations of others, by eliminating the "should's" from my running, I discovered that there was no need to compare myself to anyone else. I discovered that real uniqueness is being what you are, not in relative terms—not in simply being different from others—but in absolute terms, in being wholly and completely who you are.

Only after I stopped looking at others did I finally see myself. Only after I stopped looking to see where I fit in my age group as a runner and where I fit in some elaborate demographic as a person did I see that I am no more than who and what I am.

It is difficult at first to let go of the comfort of relativity and comparison. It is much easier to see ourselves as better than or even worse than, rather than accepting that we simply are.

LIVING A LIFE WITHOUT EXPECTATIONS

Living a life without expectations can make you uneasy at first. We are so adept at asking ourselves how we did that we find it difficult to just accept what was done. It takes some getting used to, this process of being ourselves, but in the end it is worth it.

In a sense we must rediscover our own childlike wisdom. We must understand that all we can do is all we can do. No more. Each of us will progress at his or her own speed. All of us will make progress, but it will be unique to each of us.

This is a difficult lesson to learn. Accepting who we are—as children, as runners, as parents, as lovers or spouses—is very hard to do. It's much easier to pretend that we are either more or less than we are. It's much easier to judge ourselves by arbitrary external standards than to develop an honest image of ourselves.

I had no business being a runner. It is pure serendipity that running is still part of my life. When I started I was sure I would find a way to fail at running. Why not? I had figured out how to fail at jobs, relationships, diets, and much more. But I haven't failed at running. In fact, it just keeps getting better.

If you've reached the point in your running where your expectations have exceeded the reality of your abilities, it may be time to rethink those expectations. Whether you've run for a month or a lifetime, something is wrong if you've lost the pleasure that running brings.

For running to be a part of your life, it must become a part of who you are. For better or worse, being a runner must be part of your definition of yourself. In your running, as in your life, there will be great days and there will be days that are not so great. There will be days when your life and your running are easy and days when they are a struggle.

The truth is, we can only be who we are. There are no expectations that we can meet other than those we set for ourselves. Running can teach us this lesson if we let it. Running can teach us to accept who we are and to challenge who we are at the same time.

Running can teach you how to be all of who you are. In time, with care and patience, you will get closer and closer to the essential you. Each step will take you further from the expectations of everyone else and closer to yourself.

Part Two

THE NEXT STEP

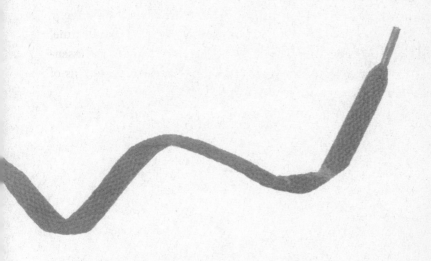

5

Becoming an Athlete

Athletes hold a special place in our culture. In exchange for their physical gifts we grant them privileges. In school, those children who display athletic prowess are set apart from the rest of us. By the time we reach high school, most of us have a pretty good idea of whether we are one of the chosen few.

My image of athletes was formed when I was a young man growing up in Chicago. It was the 1950s and '60s, when young boys played baseball—a time that many look back upon with nostalgia. It was a time for making friends, losing face, and growing up.

In those days, athletes were regarded as more than mere mortals. My larger-than-life heroes included "Mr. Cub" Ernie Banks, the tough-as-nails Bears linebacker Dick Butkus, and the late, great stock-car driver Fireball Roberts. Well, maybe Fireball Roberts wasn't an athlete, but he was a hero.

My heroes shared a love of their sport and an ability to transcend that sport. Ernie Banks was said to have loved the game so much that he would walk onto Wrigley Field and say "Let's play two!" These men were athletes playing a game with skill and determination and joy.

I learned things from these men that had little to do with baseball and football and auto racing. I learned that if you love what you're doing, if you can keep the passion alive, the journey to greatness is more important than the destination. I applied this lesson to other parts of my life, but until I became a runner, I didn't fully understand.

I also learned that athletes were different from me. The recognition they received for their efforts made my own struggles seem meaningless. Even in failure, athletes were treated with respect. If they had played well, fought hard, or simply given their all, they were rewarded with accolades. How different it was for those of us whose failures went unnoticed.

In time, those of us without athletic skills came to believe that not only were athletes stronger, faster, and more daring, they also were better than we were. Living in a young boy's world—where strength and speed and bravery were the currency of value—I felt I didn't have a dime. So from early boyhood I sentenced myself to being a spectator.

I remained a spectator for most of my adult life, contenting myself with knowing about sports and about the people who played them. I congratulated myself for understanding the sports that I enjoyed and celebrated the victories of others as though I were a participant. But I wasn't. As a spectator, I watched my own life with the same mixture of interest and detachment as I watched sporting events.

LOOKING IN THE MIRROR

All of that changed when I began to run. After four decades of standing on the sidelines, of watching others, of being a face in the crowd, I stepped into the arena. For better or worse, I chose to become an athlete. It is a simple choice, really, and one that you can make today.

How? By refusing to concede that the joy and recognition you see athletes receive is for them but not for you. You can become an athlete by choosing to use your body, whatever that body is, as an instrument of self-expression and self-growth.

In the running lexicon, the word "Penguin" has come to mean a person who runs more for the joy of running than for recognition and public rewards. Penguins are most often, though not always, found in the back of the pack at races or waddling around their neighborhoods. Some of us are perpetual Penguins. We are consumed by the pleasure of movement.

Other Penguins find their joy in the challenge of reaching their own potential, whatever that is. For some it has meant running the Boston Marathon, the only U.S. marathon that has qualifying standards. For others, it has meant finding an independence and freedom in their daily runs that expands their limits.

Can there be such a thing, then, as a Penguin athlete? Or an athletic Penguin? You may think that the phrase is a bit of an oxymoron. If your images of athletes are based on your childhood memories or the distorted images of athletes you see in the current media, being a Penguin athlete probably *is* an oxymoron.

Can people who are fighting to lose thirty or forty pounds be athletes? Of course they can! Can people who have waited until their forties to become physically active be athletes? You bet. Can people who finish last in a race be athletes? Yes, they can. And yes, they are.

For a long time, *I* thought that being a Penguin athlete was an oxymoron. Even now, when I look in the mirror, I have a hard time seeing an athlete. No amount of training, it seems, can shake my image of an athlete as someone other than myself.

I know better, of course. I am an athlete by definition. My resting heart rate, my overall level of conditioning, my shelves filled with running magazines, and my refrigerator covered with race numbers make me one. I am an athlete because my running shoes don't last six months, while my ties last a lifetime.

But meeting all of these objective criteria doesn't help convince me that I am the same as the athletes in my memory. Knowing that I engage in an athletic activity doesn't make it any easier to believe that I am an athlete. Even knowing that others consider me an athlete doesn't help.

CHANGING OUR DEFINITIONS

Something fundamental in our definition of who we are has to change before most of us can think of ourselves as athletes. Those of us who have come to running later in life first must erase years of mental tapes of ourselves as everything except athletes.

By continuing to view yourself as a non-athlete or non-runner you miss the opportunities to find joy in association with your activity. When you hear people talk about athletes or runners, it's important that you permit yourself to be included. Athletes can't be *them*. Athletes must be *us*.

Part of the problem is finding a definition of athlete in which we can comfortably place ourselves. As one who is chronically and persistently at the back of the pack in races, I can't use winning as a part of my criteria. To become an athlete, to eventually *be* an athlete, a Penguin must find his or her own definition.

Deciding what you are and who you are is never an easy matter. For example, I spent most of my life as a musician, or rather, I spent most of my life as a trombone player. Every now and then someone would try to make the act of blowing air through pipe sound more glamorous than it is by calling me a trombonist. But I was a trombone player. I knew I was because I played the trombone.

Was I a musician? That question was not as easy to answer. I had ample evidence that I was a trombone player, just as I have that I am a runner. I had the instrument, programs that listed me as a trombone player, and years of professional employment to help me identify myself as a trombone player.

As I've continued to run, I have had less and less trouble allowing myself to believe that I am a runner. I can tell myself that I am not a very good runner, or I can tell myself that I am not a very fast runner, but it has become increasingly difficult to tell myself that I am not a runner.

But accepting that I am a runner doesn't bring me any closer to seeing myself as an athlete than working as a trombone player brought me closer to accepting that I was a musician. In the purest sense, both as a runner and as a trombone player, the activity defined only what I did, not what I was.

At some point in my music career I passed from being a trombone player to being a musician. I truly don't know when or where that happened. It wasn't a particular occasion or event. It wasn't that I suddenly achieved something more than I had previously accomplished. It was more like passing through an invisible veil. On one side of the veil, I was a trombone player. On the other side, I was a musician.

After years of practicing and performing, after struggling with the limitations of my instrument and my talent, I realized that I had come to see the world differently. It wasn't that the world had changed, but rather that how I viewed the world had changed. I was looking at the world through the eyes of a musician. I was hearing the world through a musician's ears.

More important, music was no longer something I did. It was something I was. There was no longer a distinction between the activity in which I was engaged and who I was. I was always a musician, even when I wasn't playing the trombone.

There's very little question now that I am a runner. How do I know that? I'm a runner because I run. It's simple Cartesian logic. I run; therefore, I am a runner. Even for the terminally dim-witted like me, it's difficult to ignore the straightforward conclusion that someone who runs is a runner.

Like most runners, I have evidence. I have proof. If anyone were to challenge my right to call myself a runner, I would produce my running log. "See?" I would proclaim. "I ran this many miles last week and that many the week before. I am a runner."

If challenged, I could easily defend this definition of myself as a runner. As I accumulate miles, as I accumulate race numbers, as I look further back in my life and still see running, I confirm for myself that I am a runner. But am I an athlete? There still is no easy answer.

HOW YOU ENCOUNTER THE WORLD

By now, I trust that you see that being an athlete, like being a musician, is more than simple logic. Being a musician is a way of encountering the world. It is a way of encountering sound. The difference between what I hear in a Mozart symphony and what a non-musician hears is not the notes. The notes are the same—the same frequencies, the same durations, the same decibel level. What separates my experience with music is that the sounds I hear are inside of my world, not outside of it.

The same transformation occurs when one becomes an athlete. Part of the problem is that the experience of being a musician, or of being an athlete, cannot be quantified. It can only be qualified. Being an athlete is not about miles run, or times, or personal records. Being an athlete is about how you encounter the world.

Life as an athlete is very different. As dramatic as it was to go from being a confirmed couch potato to being a runner, the metamorphosis from non-athlete to athlete was even more remarkable.

It turns out that being an athlete is more than physical sensations, more than tighter muscles and a lower resting heart rate. Being an athlete is a whole new way of encountering the world around you. Being an athlete is having a body that is a tool of exploration instead of a place of imprisonment.

This was an amazing discovery for me, and for many others I'm sure. Understanding that one's body is something that can be used, that can be pressed into service as something other than a passive vessel that contains your vital organs, is a revelation of the first magnitude. Your body can become a partner to your dreams.

For non-athletes, the sensations of effort—the pounding heart, the burning lungs, the fatigue—are viewed as warning signs. In many cases they *are* warning signs. As one gets farther and farther away from any kind of conditioning and fitness, those physical sensations of effort become almost constant companions.

As a non-athlete I sought out every possible alternative to avoid effort. I paid whatever price was necessary to be able to exert myself as little as possible. For me, the sensations of effort were threatening, even frightening. As a non-athlete, I wanted to stop what I was doing and rest at the first signs of exertion and the first bead of perspiration.

As an athlete, the same sensations are the first indication that something very good is starting to happen. Feeling the sweat beginning to moisten my skin, feeling my lungs reaching for air, feeling my muscles struggling against the limits of my abilities are the sensations that I savor. Every step becomes an explosion of joy.

The very sensations that I once worked so hard to avoid are now the very sensations that I seek. Once I regarded these sensations as threatening; now I see them as a reward.

The good news, as George Sheehan said, is that we are all athletes; the only difference is that some of us are in training and some are not. We all have the capacity to live in an athlete's body and to encounter the world as an athlete. At the center of our being, we are all athletes.

EFFORT—THE MAGIC ELIXIR

The first step to becoming an athlete is changing the way you view effort. For the athlete, effort is not to be avoided; it is to be sought out. Times of effort, even extreme effort, are to be cultivated and nurtured. Moments of ultimate effort are to be celebrated. There is nothing quite as satisfying as giving all one has to give.

Effort is the fire that hardens our bodies and tempers our souls. It is a magic elixir. As athletes, we use effort like a seasoning in our lives. We mix together ingredients of effort and release in perfect proportions.

As athletes, the sensations of effort are at the very center of our world. Without those sensations, without the sweat and fatigue, our lives would be dismally ordinary. Without effort on a regular basis, our lives as athletes would become indistinguishable from those of non-athletes.

The sensations of effort, the relentless confrontation of our abilities versus our desires, are defined by us, are caused by us, and ultimately belong to us. We own those sensations in a way that we can own nothing else. In time, we not only own them, we become them.

As athletes, the sensations of effort are not outside of us; they are by definition inside of us. Effort is not something we simply observe in others. It is something we experience for ourselves. Through effort we are transformed from spectators into participants.

The sensations of effort are there at any pace, at any distance, at any age. Looking back on my first day as a runner I realize that I was an athlete even then. Even on that first run, during those first twenty-five yards of effort, I was an athlete. In that moment I chose to feel what I was feeling.

As my ability to run increased, as my ability to cover more ground on a given day increased, so did my desire to find the limit of effort that would bring on the feeling of exertion. As my pace began to get faster, I always sought out the pace that would make my body work.

BEYOND THE EDGE OF COMFORT

At any level, the purest form of effort is just beyond the edge of comfort. It is, for all athletes, that point at which they no longer are certain that they are in control. Being an athlete means pushing to the edge of uncertainty and constantly looking just beyond your capabilities.

It doesn't matter if you are a runner in the first week of training or an Olympian in the middle of a race. The search is the same: to find that point just beyond what you think your body can do. For us as athletes, the goal is to learn to live on that edge.

That edge is easy to define and impossible to find. Most of us know only that we've gotten to the edge after we've stepped off the cliff. Part of the learning process is to get closer and closer to the edge without falling off.

If you run the same route every day, in about the same time, the edge may be trying to be one minute faster when the most your body can manage is being thirty seconds faster. The edge may be trying to pass just one more runner before the finish line. That last runner may be standing just over the edge.

What often is forgotten is that the edge is different for each of us and, in fact, can be different on different days. Part of becoming an athlete is learning to accept the natural rhythm of our abilities. There are days when what was easy is hard and days when what was hard is easy.

An athlete knows this. An athlete rejoices in the easy days and accepts the difficult days. Newer runners are often at a loss to explain either the good or the bad in their runs and races. They know that one day fast is slow and that the next day slow is fast, but there seems to be very little correlation between what they do and how they feel.

An athlete accepts the cyclical nature of his or her own development and that the body is adjusting at its own rate. An athlete doesn't push past the point of adaptation. An athlete understands that the line between improvement and injury is often very narrow and walks that line with caution.

An athlete also knows that the line between honest effort and exhaustion keeps moving. My first run wasn't even a quarter of a mile. Now I can run a marathon (26.2 miles) and feel great. That doesn't mean I belittle my earlier accomplishments. Nor does it mean I believe I have achieved all that I am capable of achieving.

Being an athlete means living in a state of constant evaluation. When one becomes an athlete, one can exchange criticism for assessment. There are no bad runs or races, only episodes and events to be considered.

Being an athlete means understanding that you must always be ready to think the unthinkable. As you continue to achieve the unachievable, as you do the undoable, you must always be ready to think a grander thought and dream a grander dream.

As an athlete, when you least expect it, you may find yourself standing on the threshold of an accomplishment so monumental that it strikes fear into your soul. You must stand ready, at any moment, to face the unknown. You must be ready to walk boldly through the wall of uncertainty.

From the first day that you accept yourself as an athlete, you will have opportunities to succeed beyond your wildest imagination. The day you cover your first mile or run for an hour or finish your first marathon, you can seize the joy of being an athlete.

And when you surpass your dreams? What then? You move on. Being an athlete is a journey. It is an odyssey of discovery. And it can be the trip of your life!

6

Runner's High

One of the great mysteries of running is the thing called a runner's high. I'm a child of the '60s, and in those days being high had an altogether different meaning. At least I think it did. In those days, lots of people were high who had never run a step in their lives.

Some people have tried to explain the science of a runner's high. They say it has something to do with the release of endorphins (whatever *they* are), that the runner's high is related to morphine, and that in time runners can become just as addicted to the high from running as to any other drug. Maybe. But I don't think many of my friends from the '60s would be convinced.

I've come to think that the runner's high is more like the runner's Bermuda Triangle. We're pretty sure it's there, and we know that lots of runners have stories about it, but we can't quite pin it down.

Some runner's tell me that they feel the runner's high in just a few minutes. Other runners tell me it takes over an hour to feel it. As best I can figure, it took me about three years to feel the runner's high. It was there for me all along, but I was too blind to see it.

I had a vague notion that it was some mystical state of mind or being in which one achieved a transcendental experience of balance and peace. But I never felt it when I ran. All I ever felt was a monumental battle between my head, which wanted to continue, and my body, which wanted to stop.

It really didn't seem to matter what I did. I never felt high. If I ran too fast, I felt tired. If I ran too far, I felt sore. On runs and in races I felt silly. I felt embarrassed. I felt like a failure. But I never felt high.

I thought I could find the runner's high by running faster. I tried and tried to find the magic in the point of exhaustion. It wasn't there. I thought I could find it by running farther. I ran and ran until fatigue stole all the joy. Still, the high wasn't there.

Part of the problem, I realized later, was that I was looking too hard for that feeling. Step after step at first, and mile after mile eventually, I kept waiting to be overcome by it. I thought there was something I could do to provoke the feeling. I thought that there was some magic combination, some magic pace or distance, that would release the flood of emotions I imagined to be a runner's high.

Every now and then I caught what I thought was a fleeting glimpse of the runner's high. I would feel a little dizzy. I would feel disconnected from my body. It turns out that those feelings were most often caused by low blood sugar (because I wasn't eating enough) or by dehydration (because I wasn't taking in enough fluids.)

I thought maybe I didn't feel the high because running didn't come naturally to me. I thought that because I had waited so long to start running I had missed my chance to feel the high. I worried that because I lacked the talent for running I would somehow be denied the rewards of running.

I couldn't even figure out how fast I was supposed to run when I was trying to get a runner's high. When I heard people talk about their training paces and their race paces, I just kept my mouth shut. They might as well have been speaking a secret language! I didn't understand what they were talking about. Maybe you don't either.

PACE AND EFFORT

Pace and effort are two favorite words of runners. I guarantee that if you get into a conversation or pick up an article about running, you will come across the words "pace" and "effort." They are extremely important training and racing concepts, but pace and effort don't necessarily have anything to do with achieving a runner's high!

Pace, in its most elemental definition, means how fast you are running. Runners talk most often about pace in terms of minutes per mile. Someone who is running a six-minute pace is completing a mile every six minutes or is running about ten miles per hour. World-class marathoners will run near or below a five-minute pace. Some of us, myself included, run marathons at something closer to a twelve-minute pace. That means the lead runners are completing 26.2 miles in less than half the time it takes a slower runner to finish.

Runners also talk about training pace, which is usually slower than race pace. It is in talking about these training and race paces that the concept of effort comes up.

Effort, in its most elemental definition, means how hard it is for you to do what you're doing. Sophisticated heart-rate monitors are now available to measure with great precision your real effort. Your real effort is measured in terms of the percentage of your maximum heart rate that you can sustain for a specified length of time.

This real effort is often contrasted with your "perceived" effort. Perceived effort is simply a measure of how hard it *feels* to you. This may vary depending on how much rest you've had, what you've eaten, how well hydrated you are, the weather (heat, cold, or humidity), etc.

The goal of training is to increase your pace while decreasing your effort. Or, viewed differently, you want to be able to go at the same pace with less effort or at a faster pace with the same effort. This is, by definition, improvement.

You actually don't need fancy gadgets to measure your effort. One of the most common rules for determining effort is the "conversation" test. Can you carry on a normal conversation without becoming breathless while you're running? If you can't, you are running too hard. Your effort is too great and you very likely are doing yourself more harm than good.

This is especially true in the first weeks and months of a running program. New runners too often think they have to pound away at their bodies to make progress. It's not true. If you can't carry on a conversation, slow down.

I often ask new runners to recite the alphabet as we run together. If you are running at the right effort, you should be able to say the alphabet without panting. Another variation, from Coach Roy Benson, is the singing test. You are probably using the right amount of effort if you can talk but cannot sing while you're running.

PACING YOURSELF

Of course, I didn't know *any* of this in the early days and weeks of my running. My training pace was whatever I could manage that day. I was pretty sure I was supposed to run as fast as I could as far as I could every day, so that's what I did. I had no idea that you actually could decide on a pace to run *before* you started to run. I simply couldn't figure out how you would know how fast you could run before you started.

But you *can* know how fast to run. You can decide in advance that your run today will be an easy, conversational pace. You can decide that what you need most is recovery, not stress. You can decide before you put on your shoes what that run is going to be like.

Have I mentioned race pace? I was astounded when I learned that some runners actually predict how fast they will run a race.

This was another area of complete mystery to me. How could they know? It turns out that they know by virtue of their training. They understand what I didn't, which is that there is no such thing as 110-percent effort. There isn't. Based on your training, there is only 100 percent. That's the best you can achieve.

Being slow and inexperienced, I usually allowed my pace to be dictated by the other runners in every race. I trusted them more than I trusted myself. I would ask people what pace they intended to run and when I found someone who looked friendly, I lined up behind that person.

The real truth is that my race wasn't exactly dictated by the other runners. Since I was often the slowest, my pace usually was dictated by the next-to-the-slowest runner. During most of my early races, I adjusted my race pace to be just fast enough so that I could always see the next-to-the-slowest runner. My biggest fear was that I would lose sight of the last runner in front of me and become hopelessly lost.

From my back-of-the-pack vantage point in large races, I could almost always see the pack winding down the road ahead of me. I would watch as, little by little, the line of runners stretched like a giant streamer ahead of me. Large races became a colorful game of follow-the-leader. Smaller races all too often became an elaborate game of hide-and-seek. When I approached an intersection on the course, I had to sprint to get there in time to see which way the other runners had turned.

LOST IN THE RHYTHM

If it was an out-and-back race course, I searched for clues about the runner's high in the faces of the people near the front and middle of the pack as they ran back toward me. That didn't help much. Those at the very front of the pack always looked really serious. Those in the middle of the pack looked even more serious. And none of them looked high.

I had all but given up on experiencing the runner's high. Then one day, without warning, it happened. For no particular reason, on a quite ordinary day, in the middle of a completely unexceptional run, it hit me. I was running. I was RUNNING! My feet were carrying me across the ground. I could feel the muscles in my legs. I could feel the air rushing in and out of my lungs. I could feel my body running. The feeling was a high like none I'd ever known!

I kept running. I was lost in the movement and the moment. I was lost in the rhythm of my feet striking the ground. For a while I looked straight down at my shoes. I was fascinated by the motion of each foot. One instant my foot was there beneath me, then it disappeared behind me, then it popped back into view and the cycle started again.

I watched my hands and arms. They were moving in perfect opposition to my legs. As my foot went forward, my hand went back. Like a steam locomotive, my arms pumped back and forth, as if they were turning imaginary wheels.

I was running! I wasn't running to anything and I wasn't running away from anything. I wasn't even running because of anything. I wasn't thinking about how this run fit into my training program or how much good this run was doing my heart. I wasn't thinking at all. I was just running.

The battle between my head and my body was still going on, but they had switched sides. On that day my body wanted to keep running, while my head said I should stop.

That day I understood that running isn't a means to an end. Running isn't a way to lose weight or get fit or lower your cholesterol. It may do all those things, but that isn't the reason to run.

EASING THE PAIN OF LIVING

Maybe people who have been runners most of their lives know exactly why and how they got started. Maybe they can trace the joy they find in running to a youthful moment when their whole life was filled with promise. Maybe for them the act of running and the feeling of a runner's high have been part of who they are for as long as they can remember.

That's not the case for me or for most of the people who come to running later in life. The reasons many of us start and continue running are not always as lofty as health and fitness. As the cynicism of age begins to replace the unrestrained hopefulness of youth, running becomes a place to which many of us retreat. Some of us start running because nothing else—not booze or drugs or a life on the edge—eases the pain of living.

If life was everything we wanted it to be, many adult-onset athletes would never have turned to any sport. If our life plan was progressing as planned, if our dreams were coming true, we might never have looked for and discovered the joy of running.

The sad truth is that some of us come to the sport of running not out of a sense of accomplishment and pride but as a last resort. We come to running after abusing our bodies and spirits. We turn to running for healing, safety, security, and nourishment.

As I come to know more runners, I am touched by the stories of what running means in their lives. Even those, maybe especially those, for whom running will never provide tangible rewards in the form of trophies find a comfort in running that has been missing in their lives. Many are running from tragedy. They truly are running as if their lives depended on it.

One such story involves a woman who started running in her mid-forties. She was twelve years or so into a second marriage and twenty-five years or so into a career that had included bouncing from job to job, following her husband.

By any measure, she was successful. She had moved up the professional ladder and had taken on increased responsibilities. At the same time, she was faced with an aging body and a tenuous marriage. Her grip on the good life, the promise of having it all, of being Superwoman, had left her empty and confused.

She started running almost in self-defense. Her husband had recently started running. She could sense the changes in him and, not wanting to be left out, she bought her own running shoes and headed out onto the roads.

She had never been an athlete of any kind. Quite the opposite. She was an intellectual, bookworm type. Quiet and shy, she came to running without expectations and nearly without hope.

The changes came slowly. She discovered that her body was really well suited for running. As the miles and the months on the roads accumulated, she found herself being transformed. As she accepted the challenges of pace and distance, she began to see herself differently. Deep inside of herself, she found a runner's soul.

She announced, almost without warning, that she was going to train to try to qualify for the Boston Marathon. It was an ambitious goal for a woman of forty-five who had been running for less than two years. But she set up a training plan and stuck with it.

Her first attempt to qualify came on a perfect day. The morning dawned cool and clear. She ran her best, but missed the qualifying time. Undaunted, she tried again on a harsh, cold, windy winter day. It was not to be.

And yet the transformation in this woman was remarkable. She discovered that she could be determined and tenacious. She found that she could set goals, stay with a program, and center her life on something as important, and as forgotten, as herself.

I know so much about this woman because she is my wife. There could not be a more profound change in any relationship than there was in ours because of her running, my running, and our running.

We have logged thousands of miles side by side, we have completed twelve marathons side by side, and we have seen the best and the worst in each other.

We are together now because, through running, we have been able to see past our images of each other, past our roles, and to understand that common ground between us. We found that through our running shoes.

RUNNING INSIDE YOURSELF

At its essence running is a very private and personal matter. When I run, the first thing I notice is my physical self. I am aware of my body. I am forced to acknowledge the times when I feel good and the times when I do not. Almost from the first step, I find that I am connected to all the subtle changes in my body. I can feel my heart begin to beat with greater intensity. I can feel my lungs begin to search for the oxygen my muscles are demanding. I can feel my feet as they strike and push and resist the ground beneath me.

You cannot escape yourself when you run. In this sense, you cannot be transported to another plane. You are running inside of yourself. Everything that you are comes with you on every run. Every step is taken with your real self, not an imaginary image that you try to project.

As the run continues, your awareness of your physical self will deepen. You will feel the blood beginning to flow with greater velocity through your body. You will feel the effort and know that the effort is yours.

Even now that I have been running for several years, I am still awkward at the beginning of every run. I have never found the secret for starting the next run at the same point that I ended the last run. Early in every run my body goes through a transition from stationary to mobile.

Eventually, my joints begin to loosen, my muscles relax, and my breathing settles into a comfortable rhythm, but those early minutes of every run are always a battle. It doesn't seem to matter that I know that I can prepare for and run marathons. It is as if my psyche hasn't gotten the message. It is as if every run is the first time I have asked my body to move itself, by itself, and for itself.

The years of sedentary confinement have left their mark on my body. The ease with which I ran as a child is forever gone. Running is often deliberate now. Running is intentional.

I recall running once in rural northern California. I was waddling along with a sense of urgency when an elderly man pulled alongside me in his car. He stopped to ask me what I was doing. Astonished at his ignorance, I announced with measured indignity that I was running. Obviously unconvinced, he looked at me with suspicion and asked: "Running? From what?"

I didn't have time to tell him from what. I didn't have time to tell him that I was running simply to run. That I was running because on that day, on that road, the thought of not running never occurred to me. I didn't have time to tell him that I was running for no more important reason than because I could. I didn't have time to describe the emotional rush that overhwelmed me when I realized that I could.

In races, the experience of being high by being in touch with my feelings can be even more intense. In races I am subject not only to the joy and effort of my own body, but I find myself infected with the joy and effort of those around me.

Running a few feet behind another person, I find myself so in tune with his body that we seem inseparable. On the rare occasions when I find someone who is willing to run at my pace in a race, I feel a bond between us that reaches beyond age and gender and ethnicity. I run with him, aware only that for this one moment in time, we are together.

RUNNING TO RUN

How amazing it was to set off on an odyssey of self-discovery without a guide, with nothing more than my body and my mind. What I was going to learn about myself would come not from a book or the words of a teacher or therapist, but from my own feet. Each step would reveal a new insight, a new thought, a new feeling.

The more I ran, the more I felt myself being freed from the shackles of a life of convenience, and the more I learned. I learned quickly that my body could be my friend or my enemy. When pushed gently, it rewarded me with speed and endurance. When pushed too hard, I suffered discomfort that, if ignored, became pain.

I learned how to be defeated, but not beaten. I learned how to admire those who were faster than me without allowing myself to believe that they were better than me. I learned that the real high was in finding your limitations and exceeding them.

How I felt about myself was no longer tied exclusively to the accomplishment of distant, arbitrary goals, but to hundreds of intermediate successes that I could experience every day. I was able to develop a dynamic definition of success that took into account the reality of the moment.

Because my definition of success was always changing, I was successful more often. On some days, I succeeded just by getting out the door for a run. On others, success was measured by how hard I pushed myself during a tempo run or track workout.

The side effect of focusing on what I was feeling was that words like "winning" and "losing" were replaced by words like "doing" and "becoming" in my vocabulary. All my old notions of failure were replaced by an evolving definition of success.

When I started to run for the feeling that running brought into my life, I discovered that today's failures often lead to tomorrow's success. Failing to meet today's goal becomes less tragic if you believe that you may make it tomorrow. If you slip a little today, you do not need to give up forever.

I also learned that my spirit was not as broken as I thought. Through running I was rediscovering courage, in myself and in others. Running was awakening the very feelings that I had tried so hard to bury. Running made me aware that the true difference between success and failure, between winning and losing, is often our willingness to be honest about what success means.

Often—digging down deep for the final two-hundred-yard kick of a 5K, for example—I unleashed an almost primal energy. When I saw the finish line ahead of me I found myself so caught up in the moment that time nearly stood still. Or at the other extreme—struggling, weary and exhausted—during a five-hour marathon, I often hit a vein of emotional strength that I thought I had abandoned years ago.

In the end, it is this state of being both inside and outside of oneself that best describes a runner's high. It is that delicious moment when you realize that, on the one hand, you know yourself better than you ever have, and on the other hand, you don't know yourself at all.

Many new runners believe, as I did, that this moment, this runner's high, is reserved for those with talent and skill. While I don't doubt that those at the highest level experience a profound satisfaction through running, I also believe that we all can find our way to those feelings.

That feeling is out there for everyone who runs. It is out there for you. You can't force it, you can't predict it, but you will know it when you feel it. You will know in an instant that running has become a part of who you are, and a part of how you are defining who you will be.

Each of us can find a way to make the act of running an end in itself, too. For me, this has meant finding a way to see myself as I really am and not be afraid. It has meant finding a way to fail and not be a failure. It has meant finding a way to experience both the best and the worst that I am and accept them equally.

So if you see me running wildly through a race, don't be worried. Don't be surprised at the sight of my persistent and plodding style. And don't expect the smile to ever come off my face.

The reason to run is to run. The reason to face the struggle every day is because, every now and then, it all works. Runners call it a high. Once you've felt it, once you've experienced the magic of moving along at your own pace in your own body, you'll want to experience it all the time.

7

The Next Step

When I started running, my goal was to be able to run a mile without stopping. Since I couldn't run more than fifty yards at a time, a mile seemed like the ultimate achievable distance. After a few months, when a mile was no longer an unthinkable distance, I set my sights on running three miles.

I measured a mile and a half away from my house and made a mark in the road. This would be my sword in the stone. If I could run that mile and a half away from my house, I would have to get back. And when I did, I would have covered three miles with my own two feet.

I didn't make it to the mark the first time I tried. I didn't make it the second or third time either. It just looked too far. And if it looked too far going out, imagine how far it would have looked coming back. Still, that mark was out there, beckoning me to run past my fear.

Eventually I pushed past the point of no return. I ran until I could see the mark. Then I ran *to* the mark. The first time I made it, I stopped for a while. I wanted to savor the moment. I wanted to celebrate—not the distance, but the victory over my self-imposed limitations.

Running back, knowing that every step was taking me deeper into unknown territory, I was overcome with an odd combination of joy and anxiety. I was happy that I was running farther than I had ever run, but I was worried because I didn't know what I would do next.

Sooner or later it happens. Sooner or later the unthinkable becomes thinkable and the undoable is done. In time, a distance that was beyond the imagination becomes routine. In time, a pace that was elusive becomes ordinary. When that happens, for better or worse, we have to find new goals.

RUNNING FARTHER OR FASTER

*F*or runners, those new goals usually come down to running farther or running faster. Both can bring new satisfactions. Both can bring new frustrations. Both can bring you to new levels of understanding about yourself and about running.

At first, I wanted to go faster. Once I could comfortably run for three miles, I wanted to see how quickly I could run those three miles. Every run became a time trial. Every run became an opportunity to set a new personal best.

It is not possible, or at least it wasn't for me, to run faster every time you run. No matter how hard I tried, there were days when going faster was easy and days when I just couldn't do it. Getting faster wasn't a smooth, linear progression. It was a frustrating series of good days and bad days.

The speed came, but at a price. When I focused exclusively on how fast I was running, I stopped noticing everything else. I ran right by some beautiful sunrises. I ran through the serenity that had attracted me to running in the first place. Being a faster runner didn't make me enjoy running any more than I had when I was slower.

So I decided to try running farther. There's an old rule in running that says in order to avoid injury you should increase your mileage by no more than 10 percent per week. This is a very sensible rule and one that I'm sure came from years of experience of runners much smarter than I. It means that if you are running ten miles this week, you should run no farther than eleven miles next week. It is a very simple, clear, precise rule. It should be easy to understand.

Of course, I didn't pay any attention to that rule. If adding 10 percent was okay for everyone else, I was sure that adding 25 percent would be okay for me.

It didn't take long for my foolishness to catch up with me. Within weeks I was hobbling around with various aches and pains. It turns out that my body really was governed by the same rules as everyone else's. I was shocked. I was normal, even average!

Armed with this new information and some humility, I began to gradually and carefully add mileage. This time it worked. My daily three-mile run became four and then five. My weekly long run moved from six to eight to ten miles. I was running farther than I ever had dreamed possible.

It's human nature, I suppose. We have a natural tendency to want to do more. Once we have achieved the first level of success, we want to be able to run faster or to run farther. Neither is right, necessarily. Which you choose often depends on your personal goals and priorities.

THE FAST TRACK

If the time you have for running is limited, it may be best to focus on higher quality workouts—that is, sessions when you run with greater effort for shorter periods of time. These often produce improvements in speed. The improvement will not occur every session or even every week, but almost all who try can see gradual improvements in their running pace.

Getting faster is most often a matter of getting more efficient. The simple physics of what you are trying to accomplish dictates that you must find as efficient a means as possible to move your weight over a given distance, using as little energy as possible.

Part of what distinguishes elite athletes from the rest of us is the degree to which they eliminate everything that doesn't contribute to the task of moving their bodies forward with speed and efficiency. I recall lumbering along the lakefront path in Chicago the day before the marathon and seeing several of the eventual front-runners lope along at twice my speed.

They looked as though they were running without effort. Not many of us will ever achieve that kind of speed or efficiency, but with care it is possible to learn to run faster. It takes time and it takes patience, but it can be done.

If you decide to concentrate on speed instead of distance, one of the best ways to reach your goal is by doing interval training. This need not be a scary concept. Nor is it beyond the capabilities or comprehension of the average runner. It is simply a matter of running shorter distances at higher speeds, then giving yourself time to rest in between the intervals.

The best place to do interval training is on a track. Most of them are a quarter mile long. If possible, find a local high school or college track. Many school tracks are unused at certain times of the day and year and most schools will permit you to train on them when school athletes aren't using the track. (If you don't have access to a track, any area where you can measure a distance of approximately a quarter mile will do.)

The first time you go to a track it can be very intimidating. It's easy to get caught up in the imagined humiliation you're going to feel if you happen to be there when the track team begins to train or the anticipated boredom of running around the track in endless loops. Go to the track anyway! You'll find there's a lot more to a track workout than running in circles, and that it's really fun to tell people about your track accomplishments.

The first time you do a track workout, your goal should be to establish a baseline for your training. It doesn't matter how fast you go. What matters is that you find a speed you can run that requires some effort, but doesn't force you to slow down.

Begin your workout with a gentle warm-up. The warm-up may be anything from a half to a full mile, depending on how far you are running daily. The purpose of the warm-up is to . . . well, warm up. It is an important part of the workout and should not be skipped. It is not the time to try to impress other runners who happen to be on the track.

After warming up, begin your intervals by running one lap at a speed that you can comfortably maintain. The key is to find a speed that you can sustain for the entire lap. It does no good to start fast, only to have to slow to a crawl before you get back to where you began.

Once you've completed the first quarter mile, record the time it took you, then stop and rest. Rest for the same amount of time that you ran. If it took you four minutes to run around the track, then rest for four minutes. It's simple.

Then run another lap, again, at a speed that requires some effort but that you can sustain. Pay careful attention to how you are feeling. How are your legs moving? How are your arms moving? Do you feel like you are bouncing up and down? Learn to observe yourself.

When you've completed the second lap, record the time again and rest. Compare the times from the two laps. Were they nearly equal? Was the first lap faster? Was the second? If the times are almost equal, do another lap after you've rested.

Compare that lap time with the previous two laps. The goal is to run as many as five intervals, while keeping the effort and the time nearly equivalent. When a lap gets significantly slower or significantly harder, it's time to quit.

After you've completed your intervals, take time to cool off. Run the same distance to cool down that you ran when you warmed up. If you get tired, walk or stroll, but cover the same distance as you did in your warm-up. Then congratulate yourself. You've just done a track workout!

Over the course of the next few weeks or months, the goal of the track workouts will be (1) to increase the number of intervals by one each week until you can do ten at a steady pace, and (2) to decrease the time it takes you to cover a quarter mile. With these workouts, you are building both endurance, as you increase the number of intervals you run, and speed, as you decrease the time needed to run each interval.

Proceed cautiously with your interval training. When done well, these workouts can be very trying on the body. One interval workout a week is more than enough for most runners. For some, it is better to do interval workouts every other week. The key to progress is to find the point where interval training helps, not hurts you.

Any number of excellent books are available that outline training strategies for improving your race times. If you find that you enjoy the routine of interval workouts, these guides can help you develop a program for running faster. It may be that given who you are and where you are in your running life, the track will provide answers in your search for improvement.

Some of the lessons to be learned about ourselves can be best learned as we push toward the edges of our abilities. The truths for which we search, about what and how much we are willing to do, can only be discovered as we continue to ask more of ourselves. The threshold of exertion is comfortable for some runners. For them, the feelings that come with pushing to the extreme limits are necessary. At whatever level they may be, the pursuit of speed and the pursuit of self may be one and the same. They need the bright light of exhaustion to illuminate their souls.

RUNNING FARTHER

For some runners, it is distance, not speed, that holds the answers. The reward comes with confronting and crossing the boundaries of fatigue. For these runners, satisfaction is measured in miles, not minutes.

Running farther almost always comes down to the long run. For those who live for the distance, daily runs are necessary, but the long run is anticipated, planned, and savored.

The long run is, by my definition, any run that is one and a half times the length of your daily run. For example, if you are running three miles a day, three times a week, your long run would begin at four and one-half miles. There may be other formulas, but for most runners, one and a half the daily run is a good place to start.

To learn to run farther, you must first learn to run slower. If running faster is about efficiency, running farther is about energy management. Running farther is a matter of taking the energy you have available to you and stretching it out over a longer period of time.

For runners who are new to longer runs, I highly recommend keeping track of the long run by time rather than mileage. If your goal is to be able to run greater distances, the focus of your training must be learning to spend longer periods of time on your feet. By recording time, not distance, you avoid overextending yourself on a day when you have the will, but not the power.

One of the best ways to increase the length of time you can run is to pick one of your daily runs and add ten minutes to that run every week. For example, if your daily run is thirty minutes, stay out for forty minutes on that run the first week. The next week stay out for fifty minutes, and the next for sixty.

When you can comfortably run for an hour on that run, it's time to hold that long run steady. The next step is to gradually increase the time of your daily runs. If you are now running thirty minutes on each of your runs, increase that to thirty-five minutes on one run each week, until all of your daily runs are thirty-five minutes long and your long run is sixty minutes. Then, increase your long run to seventy minutes and repeat the pattern of adding five minutes to your daily runs one at a time, after which you again will increase the time of your long run.

Another example of a program to increase your distance/time is:

	Sun.	Tues.	Wed.	Fri.
Week 1	30 min	30 min	30 min	30 min
Week 2	35 min	30 min	30 min	30 min
Week 3	40 min	30 min	30 min	30 min
Week 4	45 min	30 1min	35 min	30 min
Week 5	45 min	35 min	35 min	30 min
Week 6	45 min	35 min	35 min	35 min

During week 7, you would run fifty minutes on the long day, and so on. By adding just a few minutes to one run every week and then gradually adding a few minutes to each of the other runs, you can safely increase the time you are spending running.

It's important to remember that these are guidelines, not absolutes. It is *much* better to increase the time too slowly than too quickly. Runners never tell me that they got injured by being too conservative!

The important thing to remember is that the total time you run per week should never increase by more than 10 percent per week. It takes careful planning and sometimes a little juggling, but it can be done. If you want to find the joy in the long run, it takes time.

Ultimately it was running farther that proved to be the greater challenge for me. I discovered that the greater the distance, the more effect tenacity had and the less important raw talent became. As the distance increases, preparation becomes nearly the equal of skill.

THE LONG RUN, HOUSTON-STYLE

Whether you decide to focus on distance or speed, I highly recommend finding a way to do a group long run once a week. These don't have to be well organized; in fact, they are often better if they're not. The ideal long-run group should include at least one older person, one very silly person, and a few crusty veteran runners. If you can't find one in your town and want to see how it's done, make a trip to Houston.

Nearly every weekend, at Memorial Park in Houston, groups of this description meet to share their joys and frustrations, to celebrate each other's successes, and to berate each other's weaknesses. I have had the privilege of running with one of these groups on several occasions. It has changed my view of the long run forever.

For starters, no one in the Houston group has any idea how far the long run actually is, since there are no mile markers. It seems to come down to a matter of what each person needs to put into his logbook that week. Considering how many years this group has been running, not knowing the distance is clearly part of their philosophy.

Then there is the hundred-yard warm-up run to the porta-potty. This scene must be witnessed to be believed. After spending ten minutes or so gathering everyone together, after ruthlessly bad-mouthing the people who decided not to show up, and after going through an elaborate pre-run routine, this group runs at 10K pace to the bathrooms.

Eventually the group begins to make its way onto the running path, meandering through parking lots, streets, and intersections. Each section of the run is marked by a service station or convenience store. I have never spent more money on a long run than I did in Houston.

The pace is casual, the conversation lively, the camaraderie intense, and the experience satisfying. In ninety minutes or two hours or more, the group in its various permutations makes its way back to the car to the *real* training goal of the morning: breakfast at Bubba's.

This may not seem like training to some hidebound traditionalists, but I think it has become much more the norm than the beat-yourself-to-death long run. It is social, it is fun, it is running at the highest level.

THE RIGHT CHOICE

But for some runners, neither farther nor faster by itself is the next step. On some days, these runners really need to run faster. On those days, they need to "feel the burn" as they say. They need to challenge themselves to push beyond comfort in order to avoid slipping quietly into acquiescence. They need not to accept what they can do, but rather to stare honestly into what they cannot do.

On other days, how fast they run doesn't matter at all. On those days, they want to run until they feel the sweetness of fatigue. They need to keep moving their feet in rhythm to overcome the confusion of the day. Some days they need to hear their feet hitting the pavement to drown out the noise of their conscience. On those days, they want just to run until they can't run anymore.

The next step? We all have to choose. We have to choose on a daily basis. And the greatest joy comes in being enough of a runner to make that choice.

8

Finding the Balance

The older I get, the more important the lessons I learned as a child seem to be. With each passing year I become more convinced that solutions for the most complex adult problems—from health and fitness and relationships to living a decent life—can be found in the stories of childhood.

The lessons taught through these children's stories are timeless, and, as it turns out, ageless. The wisdom of the tales of my youth has become more apparent as I have realized that through most of my life I have been confronted not by new problems, but more often by the same old problems presented in new ways.

Even the expressions that find their way into my adult language often have their roots in some childhood story. How often have I turned away from sour grapes or seen the truth in "The Tortoise and the Hare"?

Take the story of Goldilocks and the Three Bears, for example. This may be one of the greatest sets of instructions for life ever written. This elemental story contains a blueprint for living that can sustain us in adulthood.

Think about the overarching lesson of Goldilock's story. Nothing should be too hot or too cold. Nothing should be too hard or too soft. Everything should be "just right." The story is a primer on living a life of balance. It is a simple guide to moving away from the extremes, to seeking out that place where everything is "just right."

For runners, the lessons are there to be learned. As runners, we search constantly for the point where everything is just right. I have bought shoes that are too hard and shoes that are too soft. I have found myself on runs where I was too hot and on others where I was too cold. I have run too fast and I have run too slow. And of course, many times I have found that I have run too far or that I have run too short.

Trying to find the point that is "just right" is a constant concern for runners. If we run too much at any stage in our running career, we risk burnout and injury. If we run too little, we risk frustration from being unable to meet our goals. To be lifelong runners, we need to find the balance between doing enough to keep us motivated and doing more than our bodies can handle. It has to be just right.

It has to be just right on a daily, weekly, monthly, and yearly basis. It isn't a matter of finding the point of balance today and having the confidence that it will be at the same place tomorrow. As our goals change, as our bodies change, as our lives change, we have to search for that new place where everything is "just right."

This is easier said than done. Most of us believe that if a little of something is good, then a lot will be even better. Whether it's running or trying a new diet plan, nearly all of us will go from one extreme to the other before we find the balance point. When we read that there are benefits from exercising three times a week for thirty minutes, we believe that exercising six times a week will double the benefits. Like Goldilocks, if we have been exercising too little, our next step will be to exercise too much.

ACTIVITY AND REST

It takes a while to learn and to accept that a training program has two components: activity and rest. To be successful, we have to find the balance between activity and rest that is appropriate for us. No book, no chart, no friend or coach can devise a plan that is as well suited to our hopes and dreams as we ourselves can. We may be able to find general guidelines from these other sources, but, in fact, only *we* can decide what is just right.

During the activity phase, we ask our body to do things it hasn't done, or to do them longer or faster. If we are new to running, the activity phase may be as simple as making ourselves get out the door and move on a regular basis. In the early weeks and months of running, just doing something, anything physical will make enormous new demands on our bodies.

Later, as our bodies begin to adapt to the new activity level, we want to push past what is comfortable. We want to challenge ourselves. We want to feel the satisfaction that comes in doing more than we ever have. At any stage, this constant search for that which lies just beyond our abilities can be a potentially dangerous mind-set.

Because we take great pride in counting the minutes or hours that we engage in activity or in logging the miles that we cover, we are tempted to focus exclusively on the activity phase. Because we feel so good about the days that we engage in activity, we can easily come to see those days as the only ones that matter.

The result is that we often ignore the need for rest. The rest phase, those days when we don't run, is seen as wasted opportunity. It is torture to take a day off, especially when everything is working well. Missing a day prompts a mental message for some people that they are not as disciplined or committed as they should be.

Part of the problem is that our rest days often are imposed on us by lack of time or the imposition of other responsibilities in our lives. When we miss a day of activity because we can't fit it in, we tend to view the rest phase as being unproductive. It's very hard to take pride in having done nothing.

But resting is not doing nothing. Resting is giving the body a chance to recoup, to renew itself, and ultimately to rebuild itself into a body that will move faster or farther. The rest phase is the only time that the body has to bring itself up to your expectations.

The training effect that we all want, the changes in our body's ability to handle the stress of running occurs during the *rest* phase, not the activity phase. The adaptation process takes place while you are resting. The days when you don't run are the days when your body incorporates the new strength needed for the next run.

THE POINT OF EQUILIBRIUM

How do we find that point of balance? How do we decide what is "just right" today or this week? It's not easy. It's possible to spend a lifetime alternating between too much and too little. It's possible to search in vain for that point where your running feels "just right."

As I considered the point of balance for myself, I was reminded of a quote from *Zen and the Art of Motorcycle Maintenance* by Robert Pirsig. He wrote: "Mountains should be climbed with as little effort as possible and without desire. The reality of your own nature should determine the speed. If you become restless, speed up. If you become winded, slow down. You climb the mountain in an equilibrium between restlessness and exhaustion. Then, when you're no longer thinking ahead, each footstep isn't just a means to an end but a unique event in itself."

What a wonderful thought. Could I really find that point where I was running with little effort and without desire? Was I really willing to let the reality of my own nature determine my speed? How would I find the equilibrium between restlessness and exhaustion? And if I found it, how would I keep it?

I began to think about the formal dictates for my pace. At certain points of my running year I wanted to work on being faster. Getting faster required that I train faster. I began to consider how I decided how fast I would run on any given day. I looked at my logs to see if there was a pattern. I tried to find the objective reasons for deciding that today I would run fast and tomorrow I would run slow.

I began to think about the formal dictates of my daily and weekly mileage. At certain points in my running year I needed to increase my mileage so I could acheive a particular goal. Was I logging base miles or honing my skills for a particular race? Was I doing my long slow run or a tempo run today? Was I running the miles to meet my goals or was I meeting my goals by running the miles?

I found only a collection of rules for being a better runner or a faster runner or a runner who could run farther. I had become nothing more than a composite of training templates and programs. My logbook, not the reality of my nature, was determining my speed. I believed that every run must be one of great effort. I found that I was indeed restless and exhausted.

In the early stages of my running, the answer to the question "How fast should I run?" was easy. As I have matured as a runner, the answer has become more difficult. At first, I always ran as fast as I could—every time I put on my shoes. I never considered the reality of my nature. I only considered the reality of my slowness.

To get faster, which was my goal, I ran as fast as I could as far as I could every chance I got. As I was able to run faster, I did. All of the time. I thought that was what runners did. It was as if I was afraid that overnight I would forget how to run.

And I worried all the time about how fast I ran. I calculated the exact pace needed to run as far as I could in the time I had. If I had only an hour, I ran as fast as possible to cover as many miles as possible—as if by running more miles I would be more of a runner.

It was only much later, as I began to understand more about myself and about running, that my answer to "How fast?" changed. It was only later that I allowed myself to look at the reality of my own nature to find the speed I needed for that day. And it was only later that I understood that the search for the reality of my own nature would be much more difficult than the search for speed.

As I found that reality, I discovered that I could allow myself to run as fast as I needed to. I started every run not with a precise plan, but with a question. What is real in my life today, and what do I really need from this run? Like Pirsig on the mountain, when I start with that question, I find that how fast I run is always somewhere between restlessness and exhaustion.

By giving myself permission to be myself, rather than a dot on a training graph, I discovered it became much easier to find the point of equilibrium. By giving myself permission to be the runner I am every time I run, I found that the answers to the questions "How fast?" and "How far?" were obvious. I simply ran so that every footstep was an end in itself, not a means to an end.

THE LANGUAGE OF OUR BODIES

How do we find that balance? How do we, like Goldilocks, find the point that is "just right"? How do new runners know when they are doing more than they should? How do experienced runners know that they have gone beyond training? It's easier than you think. We listen to our bodies.

Our bodies have a built-in system for telling us when we have done too much. It took me years to figure this out, but now that I have it seems remarkably simple. When we have pushed our bodies beyond what they are ready for, we experience pain. It's as simple as that.

Pain, or aches, or tired muscles, are the body's way of communicating with our brain. When the brain decides to double the weekly running mileage in order to become a better runner, the body sends a message in pain. When the brain decides to run too far or too fast, the body reacts with pain.

Pain is the language of our bodies. When listened to attentively, the body whispers that we have done too much. If we ignore the first gentle warnings of discomfort, the body speaks more forcefully. And if we are deaf to our body's messages, the result is injury and setback.

For a long time, I thought that being in pain was a sign of progress. Pain was a source of pride. When I hobbled around on achy knees, when my muscles were so sore that I couldn't walk up and down stairs comfortably, when I was so stiff that it took me five minutes to get out of my car, I thought it meant I was getting in shape.

But you can't conquer pain. You can't control it. You can't even negotiate a peaceful settlement with pain. You only delay the inevitable. Once the pain takes over, all your strength, courage, determination, and tenacity will not carry you one more step.

I didn't realize that by working too hard I was actually working against myself. By not giving myself enough rest time, by not allowing my body to recover and adapt, I actually prevented myself from improving. The harder I worked, the less I rested and the more frustrated I became. It is a vicious cycle that is easy to fall into and hard to escape.

GETTING IT "JUST RIGHT"

Like Goldilocks, finding what is "just right" is ultimately a game of trial and error. Some days or weeks we train too easy. Others we train too hard. Neither will get us to our goals. And, like Goldilocks, the real satisfaction comes when we find the balance between too hard and too easy.

The point of equilibrium, of balance between restlessness and exhaustion, is there every day. It is not, however, always at the same place. What is "just right" today can be too much tomorrow. What brings the satisfaction of feeling "just right" changes as we change. The only constant about the balance point is that it changes.

Most runners discover that as they run for more years, as they make more mistakes in their training, and have more successes in their running, the point of equilibrium is dictated more by their state of mind than by their state of fitness. Nearly all of us find that the reality of our training year and race schedule is no match for the reality of our nature.

You will find that there are days when you will need to run with great effort to achieve the balance. You will need to know that you are capable of demanding more from yourself. You will need to know that you can push past comfort. You will need to overcome your fear of complacency. You will need to overcome yourself.

To do that, to feel at peace, there will be times when you need to feel your lungs burn and your legs ache. You will need to feel as though you can't go any faster, and then you'll dig deeper and pick up the speed. On those days you'll need to hear the wind rushing past your ears. You'll need to hear your heart pounding, letting you know that you are alive.

On other days the point between restlessness and exhaustion will be at the very edge of your abilities and will. It will be at the intersection of what you wish you could do and what you believe you can't do. At that point you must allow yourself to stop thinking and to just start feeling. It is then that you will be standing precariously at the edge of reason. It is not a place that you will want to travel to very often.

There will be other days when you will just need to run the miles—to move forward at whatever pace. You will need to feel your body in motion and know that every step is carrying you away from other people and responsibilities. On those days the real restlessness is not in your body, but in your soul. Speed alone will not separate you from yourself.

And there will be still other days when the mountain seems too high to climb, when you cannot find the desire to push yourself to your physical limits. On those days you cannot bear to think of physical pain. On those days the pain of your spirit and the weight of your angst will be all that you can carry.

All you can do on those days is to keep putting one foot in front of the other, to prove to yourself that you can. Each step will take you away from those who would have you stop. On those days you are running away. You are running to escape. On those days, the more miles you run, the harder it will be for your life to find you.

What matters most on those days is knowing that you are in control of your pace and, for that moment, your life. Running can allow you to know that, for a few minutes or hours, your life is your own. Running can allow you to stop being what you are to everyone else and find out who you are to yourself. Running can allow you to find the reality of your own nature. Running will allow you to find yourself.

Even if you've run for a lifetime you may never know for sure how fast or how far you will have to run on any given day to achieve that equilibrium. You will never know with any certainty when you will reach the point where everything feels just right. Despite a detailed training plan and goals and races, most days it comes down to looking inside and asking your soul how fast and how far you need to run today.

Like so many other lessons I've learned from running, I'm beginning to see that this equilibrium between restlessness and exhaustion can be achieved in my non-running life as well. I'm beginning to understand that I don't need to test my emotional limits every day. I'm beginning to look inside myself for the emotional pace I need that day.

I have become a Goldilocks in a world of bears. I have found that some people are too hard and some are too soft. Some jobs are too easy and some are too difficult. Some situations are too hot and some are too cold.

Through running I am beginning to see more clearly the reality of my nature. I am learning that if I become restless, I need to speed up. More important, I am finding that if either my body or my spirit becomes winded, I need to slow down.

Through running we all can find that balance. Through running we all can learn to climb the mountain of our life in an equilibrium between restlessness and exhaustion. And, with practice, we can learn that by not thinking ahead, each footstep, each run, each day isn't just a means to an end but a unique event in itself.

Part Three

THE ROAD TO VICTORY

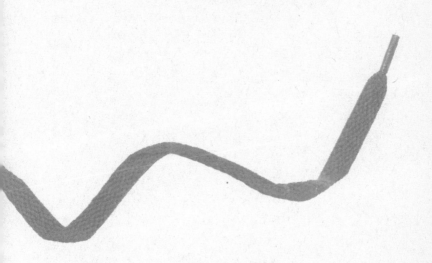

9

The Starting Line

I run because I want to. I run because through running I am discovering parts of myself that I didn't know were there. I run because most days it feels good to move my body with my own strength and will.

I race because I have to. I think most runners do. Racing on a regular basis—racing every distance from the 5K to the marathon—keeps us honest. Racing keeps us from falling into the trap of self-delusion. Racing reminds us that, like Popeye, we are what we are, and that's all that we are. Once the starter's gun is fired, there's no pretending.

Beyond that, for me, racing has also become a metaphor for life. Racing is the tangible expression of the vagaries of my existence, of the precision of my preparation as a person and as a runner, and of the simple truth that sometimes things go right, or wrong, when you least expect it.

Racing has helped me understand my place in the world of runners and in the world at large. In every race there are those who are more talented, those who have greater physical gifts, and those who have less. At every race there are those who have prepared with greater care, who have mined the limits of their talent more completely than I have, and those who haven't.

Without much effort, even beginning runners can take the

lessons learned from racing and apply them to the rest of their lives. In races, you learn to accept the unevenness of the human condition, the extent to which some people can exploit their gifts, the sheer exhilaration of a day when events conspire to create a perfect experience, and the transitory quality of those times when everything seems to go right, or, when it all goes wrong.

Like each new day, each starting line is filled with potential. For a moment, only that moment counts. Your last race means nothing. Each starting line holds the promise of greatness, even if that greatness is relative. It holds the secret to some mystery in your running life. It reveals what you are doing right and what you could be doing better.

Some runners never race. Some are content to run for their health, both physical and mental, and never feel the need to be a part of an organized race. I applaud their dedication to the activity of running, but a part of me wishes they would consider the additional joy that comes with the celebration on race morning.

MY FIRST RACE

I had been running for about six months when I competed, if that's the right word, in my first race. I had finally reached the point where I could actually run for three miles without stopping.

I knew I was getting faster. At first it had taken me over forty-five minutes to run three miles. Now I was able to run that distance in closer to thirty-six minutes. On a good day, when everything worked, I could do my favorite three-mile run in under thirty-five minutes. So, when a friend suggested a race, I was enthusiastic. I was sure I was ready.

The invitation to my initial race was extended by a man who had finished over seventy marathons and competed in nearly as many triathlons, including the famed Ironman triathlon in Hawaii. This was a man for whom racing was synonymous with life.

That first race wasn't just any race either. My friend suggested that we race in a duathlon. Of course, I had no idea what a duathlon was. He explained that it was simple. You ran three miles, rode your bike eighteen miles, and then ran three more miles. It sounded perfect to me! I *knew* I could run three miles, I was sure I could bike for eighteen, and then, since my legs would be rested from the bike portion of the race, I figured running three more miles shouldn't present a problem.

Without reservation I agreed to do the race. All I needed to know was how to go about qualifying. After all, I was from a motor-sports background in which there were categories, classes, and qualifications. If I was going to race I would need to meet the qualifying standards.

I was shocked when my friend Lee said I was already qualified, that all I needed to do was show up and pay my entry fee to receive a race number. He patiently explained that in the sport of running a rank beginner gets to compete against the very best. I knew immediately that I was going to like the sport of running as well as the activity itself.

That first race morning I was filled with expectation, trepidation, and a desperate lack of preparation. When I arrived, the other competitors had already begun their warm-up routines. Undaunted, I unloaded my bicycle, made my way to the registration table, paid my entry fee, and began my career as a racer.

Not knowing anything about the sport, I did my best to imitate those around me who seemed to be more experienced. I watched what they did and tried to do the same. When they stretched, I stretched. But people were stretching parts of their bodies that I didn't think I had. When they ran, I ran. By the time I got to the starting line I was already exhausted.

As the competitors began to gather at the starting line, I made my way into the front row. After all, I didn't want to give anyone an advantage. I knew I was running much faster than I had six months earlier. I knew that sometimes I was running nearly an eleven-minute-per-mile pace, so I was *sure* I would be competitive. As I took a place in the front row, I wondered if the other competitors were aware that there was a new kid in town.

Then Lee tapped me on the shoulder and announced we wouldn't be starting in the front row. I complained briefly, but conceded that perhaps there was a protocol that was unknown to me in this sport. Grudgingly, I moved back to the second row.

Lee tapped me on the shoulder a second time, quietly explaining that we weren't going to start in the second row either. I was outraged. Why not? I was there to race. I was there to race to win! How could I expect to win if I kept giving ground before the race began? Indignantly I asked him where we were going to start.

Calmly, Lee answered: "We're going to start at the back, with no one behind us." Of course, it's a good thing we did, because that's exactly where we finished. At the very back, with no one behind us.

I learned some very important lessons that day. I learned that thinking only in terms of my own improvement had little to do with how I would fare in the real world of racing, that a race can be a long and sometimes discouraging affair. And I learned that there is something magical about seeing the finish line.

I *did* finish. I even managed to finish with a certain flair, raising my arms in victory as I crossed under the finish-line banner. In mock Olympic victory style, I celebrated with the enthusiasm usually reserved for world champions. I celebrated victory over myself, my fear, and my ignorance.

I knew I was hooked as soon as I finished, that racing was going to become a part of my life. I knew I would be much more willing to train and to test my limits if I had a venue like racing through which I could see the truth about what I was and what I wasn't.

For many runners, the first race is an exercise in anxiety and worry. It needn't be. As new racers, we worry most about what others will think of us. Will we be too slow? Will we be embarrassed? Worst of all, will we finish *last?*

As one who has finished last, I can tell you that it isn't that bad. It may be a little nerve-racking to have a police car or ambulance trailing you, but the sensation of finishing and the emotions that come with crossing the finish line are just as powerful for the last finisher as for the first.

HOOKED ON RACING

I was hooked on racing. And that meant training, so I trained. Like many adult-onset athletes, I had no idea what training meant. I had never been on a team, never had a coach, never had a conversation with anyone about how to train.

But I wanted to improve, so I did what I could to get better. I bought books on how to get faster and how to train smarter, be stronger, and win the mental and physical game of running. I followed the recommended plans as best I could. Unfortunately, the charts never showed the pace that I was running. I was slower than the slowest charts. Still, I was training.

In time I raced again. I had trained hard and I had improved. I had increased the distance I could run and decreased the time it took me to run it. I had the mind-set of a racer. I was a lean, mean, racing machine! At least I was in my own mind.

My second race was also a duathlon. This one seemed easier, though, because you ran five miles first, then biked twenty-five miles. There was no second run. What a relief! I wouldn't have to face a second run on tired legs. This would be fun!

Somewhere on the application form for the race, I noticed that it was a qualifying event for the World Duathlon Championships. I had no idea what that meant, but I thought that it would at least provide me with some competition. I was *much* better than the last time I had raced, after all.

Standing at the starting line again, I was ready. I positioned myself in the middle of the pack this time, keenly anticipating the start. My heart was pounding. I knew this was going to be my day. This was going to be the day the racing world took notice.

At the command of "go" the pack of runners around me disappeared. In the time it took to glance down to start my watch and look back up, everyone else had taken off. With the exception of my wife, who was also racing for the second time in her life, I was alone. I was alone, in shock, and dead last.

I bolted down the course. With Karen in tow, I ran as fast as I could go. By the end of the first mile I was completely exhausted and still losing ground. I had run the fastest mile of my life, in just under ten minutes, and was by far the slowest person in the race.

My reaction was to start to laugh. The man calling out the time at the first mile marker was startled to see me so far behind and laughing. I'm sure he thought I was crazy, or stupid, or both. It didn't matter. I was last, I was slow, and it was funny.

I laughed mostly at my own ignorance and my arrogance. I knew so little about the sport that I had allowed myself to believe I could be competitive. I knew so little about the talent and dedication of the other competitors that I believed I could beat them. I was last, I was slow, and I was just beginning to see myself for the first time.

It was as close to a flash of enlightenment as I have ever had. In that instant I realized that my best was not good enough. I realized that I was not going to undo the damage I had done to my body in a matter of months or even years. I realized that if I was going to stay in the sport of running, I would have to find a reason other than winning.

STANDING AT THE STARTING LINE

I have now stood at the starting lines of hundreds of races with thousands of runners. I have never won. I have raced with runners who have run years longer than I have who also have never won. And I have learned from them that, for many, the victory is, indeed, in getting to the starting line.

In most of our lives there are very few times when we are required to be completely honest with ourselves and with those around us. We spend thousands of dollars to make ourselves look better or seem smarter or richer than we really are. Someone once told me that for most of his life he had worked a job that he didn't like so that he could buy things he didn't need to impress people he would never meet.

Standing at the starting line, the illusions we use to create ourselves are useless. No amount of money or status, real or perceived, means a thing once the race starts. For better or worse, the starting line is the true source of equality. In the middle of a race, when you are giving all you have to catch another runner or digging down to keep from being overtaken, there are no age or gender or race differences. There is only another runner.

Those who run but never race are missing out on a great celebration, too. Standing with 16,000 other runners at the beginning of the Marine Corps Marathon, for example, is a feeling that must be experienced to be understood. Standing there, with so many other runners who share a common goal and a common dream, is a powerful affirmation of our own goals and dreams.

More than that, standing at the starting line is the time when we can see ourselves most clearly. The starting line is where we can experience the enigma of life—that we are each alone and yet part of a larger group. Standing at the starting line we see those around us as both competitors and companions. We see them, as we can see ourselves, as people with an inescapable need to be part of some-thing outside of themselves, while still maintaining the integrity of who they are.

It is a strange sensation to know that we are both the same as, and distinct from, those around us. We look alike, we're dressed alike, and yet we are completely unique. It is also unsettling to re-alize that what you are feeling is shared almost exactly by the per-son next to you. And it is not always easy to reconcile the emotional paradox that those around you are your competitors while also be-ing those with whom you have the most in common.

Beginners can experience the same feelings as veteran runners. It isn't a matter of how long you've been a runner, but of how you al-low running to inform your life. If you are open to the lessons of racing, every starting line can be a seminar in becoming yourself.

These lessons can occur at any distance. A 5K race (3.1 miles) is more than long enough to discover the truth. A 10K race (6.2 miles) doesn't guarantee twice the revelation, but it gives you more time to reflect. And distances beyond the 10K—15 and 20Ks, half-marathons, the full marathon—are out there if the answers are buried so deep within you that mining for the truth takes longer.

WHY I RACE

Many experienced racers have told me there was a moment when all their feelings about running and themselves crystallized. That happened during a particular race for me. In one fleeting mo-ment, all the reasons I race came into clear view.

I was entered in a 10K (6.2 miles). I like 10Ks. They are long enough to require preparation, a taper, and a race strategy, but short enough that I can walk normally the next day. I like them because, with a decent training program, even the terminally sluggish like me can show improvement.

I had run most of my previous 10Ks in about an hour. In some races I had run just under an hour and in others I had struggled to finish in an hour and ten minutes, but I had been training hard and focusing on this particular race. I was determined to set a PR (personal record).

The day couldn't have been better for racing. It was a cool morning. The crowd was large enough to generate enthusiasm but small enough not to impede the runners. I lined up farther forward in the pack than I normally did. I was prepared to lay it on the line. I was going to see how good I could be.

By mile four, though, I had all but given up on setting a personal record. The opening miles had been slow by design, but I feared I had miscalculated my ability and desire. I was running consistently, yet I couldn't find the extra effort I needed. I was beginning to run down folks whose fatigue was more obvious than mine, but I was falling into a late-race melancholy.

Then I passed "him," the man who would show me how to find the best in myself. He did not appear to be an exceptional person in any way. He was average—a man about my age, height, and weight. Nothing distinguished him from the other runners. But, as ordinary as we both were, he was not content to see me waddle by. Rather than concede to me, he challenged me and passed me back. I hate that! Now I was going to have to stop feeling sorry for myself about missing a PR and race him.

So I came back up on his shoulder. Seeing that we were about to overtake another runner, I passed on the right and blocked him in. Pretty good strategy, I thought. But he just went wide right and came by me again.

I hate that!! With less than half a mile to go, my lungs were screaming for more air, my legs were feeling like they were going to fly off at the hips, and my rational self was explaining to my running self that this was *really* dumb. Nevertheless, I summoned what reserves I could muster and pretended to effortlessly pull away.

The last three hundred yards were on a quarter-mile track. Fearing that he would catch me again, I pressed on. Rounding the final turn I could see the clock. I was going to do it! I was going to run the fastest 10K of my life, and he had helped me do it.

In the finish chute, I turned to find him, but he was nowhere to be found. Somewhere in the last half mile I had dropped him. I never did see him finish, and I never had the chance to thank him.

The truth was that for a few minutes he was the most important person in my life. I wanted him to know that. I wanted him to know that by trying to beat him, I was really trying to overcome myself.

For those few minutes he became teacher and mentor and coach. Without saying a word, he helped me find something inside myself when I thought everything was gone. He taught me a lesson I have had a hard time learning: that there is more to me than I ever imagined.

CONFRONTING THE FEAR

No matter how long you've been a runner, it is through racing that you learn the truth about integrity. Most of us find the truth about what we are willing to do, willing to be, and willing to become at the edges of our ability. As we approach, and exceed, our expectations in races, we discover our true limits. In failing to be true to ourselves—by not exerting ourselves or by exerting ourselves too much—we reveal the essence of who we are, who we have been, and who we are becoming.

One thing that never changes, regardless of how many races I've run, is the fear. It's the fear of the unknown. It's the fear of what I may find out about myself, the fear that what's ahead is something I haven't planned for and may be unprepared for. It could be something that will force me to see myself differently.

Those of us who have come to running later in life, for whom every race is a physical and emotional experiment, eventually develop the mental attitude of a test pilot. The fear is always present, but it doesn't stop us. The fear of failing doesn't paralyze us. We don't let it.

When we confront this fear through racing, we can learn to confront it when we're not racing. We may discover, for example, that there are times when no amount of preparation is enough to overcome the unexpected in a race. We may come to see that the same is true in life. On the other hand, as we gain confidence in our ability to prepare with precision for a race, we see the value in using the same precision in preparing for life.

In the end, it comes down to honesty, to learning how to live with yourself all day, every day, without creating false illusions of competence or inability. It comes down to learning how to figure out exactly who you are, what your skills are, what the limits of those skills are, and whether there's anything at all that you can do about it.

Before I raced, I was often tempted to both over- and underestimate my abilities. In life, as in those first races, I sometimes allowed myself to believe that I was better than I really was. More often, though, I allowed myself to accept that I was much less than I really was.

Every day is like a starting line now. Every day I have to face myself with the same honesty that I do when I race. Every day I have to confront those who are more talented, better prepared, or more experienced than I. Every day I have to chose between the isolation of my world and the celebration of the world around me. And every day I get just a little better at making that choice.

10

Race Relations

Runners often are thought of as solitary individuals. The popular image of the runner, especially the long-distance runner, is of one who prefers the peace and solitude of the open road to the hustle and bustle of modern life.

When we think of runners, many of us picture an individual running alone along a deserted stretch of highway, lost in thought, carried forward by an unattainable grace and fluidity of movement. The vision we have is of a person inseparable from the surroundings, but distant from other people.

To some extent the picture is accurate. Many runners prefer their own company to that of others. Some runners only find satisfaction in running if they are alone. And, frankly, some runners just aren't very friendly. They run alone mostly because no one wants to run with them!

But the distance between runners breaks down at races. Races are the occasions when hundreds or thousands of solitary runners gather at a single spot to celebrate themselves and each other. Races are when each of us becomes all of us.

Somewhere between uniqueness and sameness is the aggregate of who we are when we become part of something beyond us. Gathering together on the morning of a race, it's difficult not to see the larger picture—the picture of ourselves as more than simply a runner, the picture of ourselves as part of a community of people who run.

At races I have found myself laughing with people I've never met. I've found myself locked in battle with people twice my age and people half my age. I've found myself cheering for people running past me. These are people who, on the surface, are better than me. They are, at least, faster than me at that moment in time.

It is only at races that I realize why I must continue to run. There I grasp most completely both my uniqueness and my sameness. At races I see most clearly how arbitrary the boundaries are between myself and the rest of the world.

THE IMPOSTOR

Most of our images of racers, whether in running or other sports, are based on what we've seen on television or in movies. The media's focus is usually on hard-edged competition, the will to win, the drive to overcome obstacles, or the persistence to press on when all hope is gone.

This romantic notion of racing prevents us from viewing ourselves as racers. The thought of "hanging it all out" is not a concept with which we are very comfortable. We've got to be able to get to work the next day, after all.

Viewing ourselves merely as recreational runners, as those who run more for pleasure than for pain, we often feel we are less than real runners. If we aren't willing to play hurt and win one for the gipper, we consider ourselves second-rate racers.

Races weren't always a time of celebration and communion for me. For several years they were a time of fear and intimidation. On race mornings I was forced to see the truth about myself, to face the things that I ignored in my training. Races were occasions to punish myself for failing to train harder or run faster. I used races to prove to myself that I wasn't any good at running.

For a long time I was embarrassed to be standing in a group of runners with a number pinned to my chest. How presumptuous, I thought, that I should try to join in. How outrageous of me to think that I, a waddling middle-aged man, could be one of them.

I remember standing at the starting line—no, actually standing well away from the starting line—when the nervous energy began to build at one race. I found myself trying to hide in the crowd, afraid that the race director would spot me, the impostor, and ask me to leave. "Hey you!" he calls out in my nightmare. "What are you doing here? This is a race for real runners!"

It never happened, of course. I was never singled out as the only non-runner. In time, I learned that rather than being resentful of my being a part of the celebration, most of the other runners were very encouraging.

Sometimes other runners would even offer advice. I tried to listen carefully as they explained their own race strategies. I even tried to look interested as they described in detail their plan for attacking a particular race course. I tried not to let them know that my only plan was to try to finish under my own power, that my only strategy was to try to stay in front of the ambulance that trailed the last runner.

I remember asking a friend for advice on how to run a 10K. I had run a few 5Ks and felt pretty comfortable with the distance, but I had not run a 10K before. He explained that my goal should be to run negative splits and that the way to accomplish that was to stay below my anaerobic threshold for the first three miles and then begin to push toward my VO2 Max as I got closer to the final 400 yards. His answer made perfect sense to him.

I looked at him, my eyes glazed over, and assured him that he had described precisely what I had in mind. I had no idea what he was talking about, but he seemed so convinced that his plan would work that I felt I had no choice but to agree. Of course, I also knew that, as soon as the gun went off, he would be so far ahead of me he wouldn't know if I had followed his plan or not.

But once I discovered the joy in racing, I raced all the time. One year I raced nearly every weekend, trying every distance I could. I'd drive anywhere to race with anyone. I couldn't get enough!

ONLY FOUR KINDS OF RUNNERS

I learned a lot that year. I learned that running negative splits means you run the second half of the race faster than the first half, that my anaerobic threshold is the point at which my legs begin to feel as if they are turning to stone, and that my VO2 Max is almost exactly the point at which I want to vomit.

I learned that the runners in the back of the pack have different things on their minds at the beginning of races than the runners at the front. And I learned that, when you get right down to it, there really are only four kinds of runners. There are the really fast runners, the pretty fast runners, the kind-of-fast runners, and the back-of-the-pack runners whom I call Penguins.

After several years of racing I can tell what kind of runner a person is before the race begins. I know in advance who will line up where in the pack. It's simple when you know what to look for.

The really fast runners are national- or even international-caliber athletes. They are the runners who have a real chance for an overall win at any race they enter. Many of these runners have names you can't pronounce.

The really fast runners don't talk to anyone before the race starts. They are deep into their warm-up routines and are making sure that the competition around them doesn't gain any physical or mental advantage. They are serious, business-like competitors.

The really fast runners always wear the same thing: running shorts, a singlet, and running shoes with no socks. It doesn't matter if the temperature is below freezing; the really fast runners still wear shorts, a singlet, and running shoes with no socks. The exception to this rule is when the wind-chill factor drops to around forty degrees below zero. Then the really fast runners put on white cotton gloves.

The pretty fast runners are the local runners who, on a good day at the right race, may have a chance at an overall win. The pretty fast runners know the names of the really fast runners, and they know how to pronounce them. The pretty fast runners annoy the really fast runners by trying to talk to them.

For reasons that elude me, it seems that the pretty fast runners are never actually competing in the race that they're in at the time. They frequently say things like: "This is just a tune-up race for me. I'm getting ready to qualify for the Intergalactic Track Team, so I'll probably just cruise the race this morning at about a six-minute pace."

My favorites, though, are the kind-of-fast runners. They are the runners who, on any given day, have a chance at placing in their age group. The kind-of-fast runners are easy to spot. They are either (1) injured right now, (2) just coming back from an injury, or (3) worried about reinjuring themselves.

Standing around with these runners is like being at a sports medicine clinic. They are wearing more devices than you can imagine for solving one malady or another. Kind-of-fast runners are always taped and Ace-bandaged together.

Finally, there are the runners at the back, the runners I call Penguins. By the time I get to the back of the pack, I know I am among friends. I know that I am around people who think the way I do, run the way I do, and worry about the same things I do.

BACK-OF-THE-PACK WORRIES

*I*n the back of the pack, we are worried about the really big issues. Will I be able to go the distance? Will there be any post-race food left by the time I finish? And most important, where are the bathrooms along the course? Those of us in the back—those who require well over two hours to finish a half-marathon or five and a half hours to finish a marathon—will definitely need to find a bathroom during the race.

At the beginning of my first half-marathon, I knew I was in trouble. I'd read about proper hydration, so I had guzzled water for days. I spent twenty minutes in the porta-potty line before the race. Eighteen of those minutes were spent standing in front of an empty porta-potty because the guy in front of me got out at precisely the same moment I turned around to wave at my wife.

And, of course, it was the one porta-potty without a lock. I was trying to use the facilities *and* hold the door closed so that the vision of me with my running shorts down wouldn't be burned inexorably into the collective memories of the other runners standing in line. Plus, I knew people were waiting in line, so performance anxiety of another sort set in.

Part of the problem during long-distance races is that because we at the back of the pack are on the course so much longer, we also consume more water over a longer period of time. I've seen the front runners come through a water table. It's like a ballet movement. They grab the cup, toss exactly two ounces into their mouths in a perfect arc, splash the remainder on their faces, and never lose stride.

Those of us in the back, on the other hand, take our time at the water tables . . . as though we're at the breakfast buffet at Shoney's. We look closely at the cups of water and carefully select the ones we want.

By the time the back-of-the-packers get to the tables, the volunteers sometimes are trying desperately to get rid of the water. So we end up drinking two cups as we pass the table, then carrying another with us. By the third water table, we definitely are looking for the porta-potties!

But, in the end, it is the slowness with which we back-of-the-packers run the race that makes the experience so pleasant. Many runners at the front have no idea just how wonderful the volunteers are, for example. They shout encouragement as we pass and stay on the course until the last runner finishes. I high-five the young volunteers and blow kisses to the older ones. And I thank every one of them.

Because I'm not in a big hurry, I have had time to get and give hundreds of smiles. For me, and others at the back of the pack, races are opportunities not only to get to do something good for ourselves, but to do something nice for other people. For many of us, that contributes to the satisfaction we get from racing.

The actual experience of racing is different for those of us at the back of the pack, too. I recall someone asking an elite runner if it was true that the real race was the race against the clock. The elite athlete gave a motivational answer about how the most important thing in races is to stay within yourself, to race within your training, and not to race against the clock.

That's well and good for those who are finishing early, but for me nearly every race is a race against the clock. All too often, I'm racing to finish before they take the clock down! For those of us who are trying to finish before the award ceremony is over, the race against the clock is very real.

As I've continued to race, I've seen and admired many really fast runners. They are truly beautiful to watch. I've actually known some pretty fast runners. Although I've never been invited to run with them. I've even been acquainted with some kind-of-fast runners, and at times have fashioned myself after them. But nearly all my friends are Penguins.

I'm not altogether sure why that is. It may be because the really fast runners talk to no one, the pretty fast runners try to talk to the really fast runners, and the kind-of-fast runners talk to themselves. At races, I end up talking to, and becoming friends with, the people around me at the back of the pack.

I've developed a system for identifying the person who will be the most interesting to run with at any given race. By using this system I am almost guaranteed of having good company and hearing a fascinating story before the race is over.

My system is this. I look for someone wearing a T-shirt from some other type of sporting event. For example, if you can find someone in the back of the pack who is wearing a professional bass fishing tournament T-shirt, I promise you he will have an interesting story to tell. He may even be running as slow as you.

It seems like every one of the racers at the back of the pack has an interesting story to tell. I have heard tales of heroism, like the couple who were running together to celebrate their victory over drug and alcohol addiction. I have heard stories of courage, like the stroke victim who dragged his left leg through an entire marathon. He had once been a pretty fast runner. The thought of being able to run again, at any speed, had sustained him through his recovery.

THEY'RE CHEERING FOR YOU

But the most extraordinary reason to race was given to me by the most ordinary of runners. He was in his mid-forties, as I was. He had been running for only a few years, as I had. He had worked hard and raised a family. He had done all the things that he thought he should do.

We were running together at the midpoint of a large marathon.

The day was beautiful and the crowds were terrific. At every turn, in every neighborhood, people lined the streets and crowded the intersections to share in the moment and shout encouragement to the runners.

I looked over during the race and saw that this man had tears streaming down his face. My first thought was that he had injured himself. I could almost feel his disappointment as I moved closer to him. From the pained look on his face, I was sure that his race was over.

"What's wrong?" I asked. "Are you hurt?" "No," he replied softly, "I'm not hurt." "Then why the tears?" I asked. "Because . . . I just realized that in my entire life, no one has ever cheered for me before." Soon I was crying with him.

This experience is possible for every runner, even for those who are finishing hours behind the leaders. Racing is your chance to be both who you are and who you want to be. At races, even the most ordinary runner gets to hear the cheering crowds. For thirty minutes or five and a half hours *you* are in the arena. When you are racing, you can allow yourself to accept the cheers and accolades that you might otherwise deny yourself. You can see yourself as the hero, perhaps for the first time.

Once you accept yourself as a hero, you can begin to understand that there are winners all along the race course. I used to believe that there could only be one winner. What a moment of enlightenment it was to discover that there are individuals who are winning races irrespective of their finishing time.

And what a moment of monumental enlightenment to discover that you are one of those winners! What a difference it makes to know that what separates those at the back of the pack from those at the front is nothing more than the time it takes to cover the course. What a change it makes in wanting to race when you finally understand that it is accepting the challenge to find out who you are on that day that makes you a winner.

At races, you can be what you hope you are. You can be strong and powerful. You can be fluid and graceful. You can discover that, when you dig down deep enough, you will find the person you've always wanted to be. Racing gives all of us the opportunity to find the best in ourselves and the best in those around us.

Running may be a solitary sport for some. But for those who have spent their lives in a different kind of solitude, races are a time to find the connectedness they've needed. At races, you can find those who share your hopes and dreams.

Standing at the beginning of a race, alone but united, you can find the quiet peace that comes in knowing that your uniqueness is shared by others. Surrounded by other runners, waiting for the race to begin, you can find a calm confidence in knowing that your individual odyssey is actually just one stone in a mosaic of self-discovery, a mosaic crafted by all those who, like you, have accepted the challenge to overcome the distance set before them, using only their bodies and their will.

11

The Finish Line

All of us, I suppose, take ourselves too seriously from time to time. I know I do. Despite my best efforts, some days it's hard to avoid thinking that I am the center of the universe. Some days I'm convinced that the world should make allowances for me. I want all traffic lights to be green. I want the line I'm in to be the fastest-moving one. I want special consideration from everyone I encounter.

If you find yourself asking the universe for too many favors, the best way to shake the feeling of self-importance is to put on your running shoes. There's something about putting on your running shoes that drags you back into reality and helps you regain your perspective.

The process of regaining my perspective usually begins with the sight of nine different pairs of shoes, all in various stages of being broken in or worn out, scattered about the floor of my bedroom. I take note of the careful matching of the numbers on my running socks. I observe, with a touch of humor, the fact that I put the date of purchase on my running underwear. I don't know what about this helps me get centered, but it does. It's true for many runners. The very act of getting ready for a run brings us back to our selves.

As we apply lubricant to every body part that may rub another body part or article of clothing and then chafe, we are forced to see our real body, not just the body of our imagination. We are required to look carefully at both the parts of that body that have responded well to the rigors of running and to the parts of that body that carry the evidence of previous indiscretions. Getting ready for a run requires us to see what we have been and what we are becoming.

As we carefully straighten the toe seams of our socks, we think about how much more important our body seems to us now. As a late-blooming runner, I think about my feet and legs and wonder how, for so many years, I could have ignored their need to move.

As my vanity prompts me to adjust my running shorts so that I'll look as trim as possible, I am buoyed by what is happening to my body and my spirit. Then, as I put on the lucky hat that any normal person would have thrown away long ago, I begin to see the folly in my vanity. As a runner, self-acceptance isn't merely a goal, it's a prerequisite.

In coming to accept myself, I am beginning to recognize even before I head out the door that despite all the training, all the racing, and all the smarter decisions about what to put in my body over the last few years, underneath it all is the same old me. Even in running shorts and shoes, I still am trying to portray an image of someone who I rarely am—someone who knows for sure what he is doing.

I realize that if I were choosing the person around whom the universe would revolve, I wouldn't choose me, or probably any other runner. I certainly wouldn't choose someone who argues the relative benefits of gel versus air versus grid. I figure if you use words like CoolMax and GU with a straight face, the center of the real universe has probably moved past you.

I can't imagine a situation in which my importance should pre-empt all others. Most of my life has been painfully ordinary. Any universe with me at its center would be hollow at its core, I think. It's easier for me to accept that when I am dressed in shorts and a singlet than it is when I am wearing a three-piece suit and power tie.

Maybe that's just as well. Being a runner often means going to the edges of our own experience and ability. That edge can be one mile or one hundred miles. It doesn't matter. What matters is not that we need to be at the center of the universe, but that through our efforts our own universe continues to expand.

THE REALITY OF THE MARATHON

When I really need help regaining my perspective, nothing works as well as a race. If I begin to think that I am too important to the fate of the universe, nothing makes me see my insignificance more than a race. Races are real. Races happen in real time on real courses with real people.

If I have indulged my ego for a long time, the race that works best is the marathon. Nothing is more humbling than the reality of that distance. If I can't find the truth in 26.2 miles, I have lost it forever. Maybe that's why I like to run marathons. Because I began the search for myself so late, I need all the time I can get to cover those 26.2 miles, to find the truth. I enjoy the time of discovery that running marathons affords me.

It's certainly not that I like marathons because I have a special gift for running them. For me, a good marathon is any marathon that I finish. And a great marathon is one that I finish in less than five hours. In the years that I have been running marathons I have had more good ones than great ones.

The marathon distance is daunting to many new, as well as to some experienced, runners. It is not a distance to be taken lightly or a training goal to be set on a lark. Nor is 26.2 miles magic—it's just that it takes some of us that long to find the truth.

Like many runners, the goal in my first marathon was to simply finish. My definition of success was crossing the finish line, no matter how or when. At least that's what I thought initially.

As my training runs got longer, as the weekly mileage began to add up, and as my body began to experience the cumulative effect of my ignorance, it occurred to me that I might need to redefine success. Success might simply be starting the marathon healthy and unhurt. To finish would be a bonus.

I finished my first marathon four hours and fifty seven minutes after I started it. With that single, final step began an odyssey of self-discovery and self-affirmation beyond my imagination. I had no idea, then, that the last step of one marathon is really the first step of the next.

Other marathons followed. Among them was a miserable run in the rain, a glorious day in the sun, a determined and painful walk of the final fourteen miles, and a sobering ride in the straggler's van. Then there was the hundredth Boston, where I walked the last six miles because I didn't want the day to end.

In fact, I don't want *any* marathon to end. That may be the problem. While other runners seem determined to get through the marathon as quickly as possible, I don't want it to be over. By the midpoint I'm thinking that I've already had half the fun I'm going to have that day, and I start to get sad. After that, it gets worse. By mile eighteen the markers seem too close together. Time is flying by. I want everything to slow down.

So I *do* slow down. Not because I'm tired or hurt, but because I don't want it to be over. By mile twenty-three the feeling is almost paralyzing. It's the strangest sensation! Once I know I'm going to finish, I don't want to.

I encourage all first-time marathoners to slow down at mile twenty. It's your first marathon and you only have one first time. I encourage marathon novices to thank every police officer and every volunteer. I tell first timers to take water from the youngest child at every water stop and to look that child in the eye and say thanks. If you take time to savor your first marathon, the others will be much more enjoyable.

Some runners want only for the marathon to end. Their satisfaction comes when they cross the finish line. I understand that, but I think they often miss much of what makes a marathon so satisfying. The last step of one marathon really does become the first step toward the next.

Sooner or later, in every marathon, I begin to laugh. There's a foolishness about marathons that is obvious to everyone except those who attempt to run them. Except perhaps for the truly gifted athletes, one must have a sense of humor about the act of running 26.2 miles for no particular reason.

My laughter begins quite early in some marathons, sometimes before the start, as people engage in their pre-race rituals. Not that my rituals are any less peculiar. Mine inevitably focus on the lines at the porta-potties. The window for the perfect pre-race porta-potty visit is very small for me. If I get in line too soon, I'll need to get back in line before the race starts. If I wait too late, pre-race nerves take over.

Out on the course, the laughter can occur anytime. At one point in the Marine Corps Marathon those of us in the back caught a glimpse of the lead runner. His fluid speed and form, in contrast to mine, underscored the absurdity of trying to compare myself to other runners. Just observing his grace made me smile.

Often though, it is only in the latter stages of the marathon that I realize the joke is on me. As the miles turn the minutes into hours, as I begin to run past the walkers and walk past the runners, the humor becomes obvious and my perspective returns.

THE TRUTH ABOUT FINISHING

Sometimes the lessons and humor come from the runners around me, as happened during the Chicago Marathon. That day a woman whose name I don't know taught me the value of humor and the power of hope.

I was leading the five-hour finishers pace group for *Runner's World* magazine. This woman and I had run together for nearly twenty-five miles. She stayed so close to me that I nicknamed her Velcro Lady. Mile after mile she stayed at my shoulder. She was determined that I would lead her to a sub–five-hour marathon.

As we took a walk break at mile twenty-five, I said jokingly that it was time to start thinking about the finish-line photo. I admonished the runners near me not to stop their watches as they crossed the line because then their faces would be hidden from the camera. I encouraged them to think about how they wanted to look in the picture.

At my suggestion, Velcro Lady got a huge smile on her face, reached down into the pocket of her running shorts, and pulled out a tube of lipstick! Lipstick!! What a story of hope. She was *so* hopeful about finishing that she carried a tube of lipstick for twenty-five miles *just* to be ready for the finish.

Unfortunately, one's motor skills are not very precise after running for nearly five hours. Velcro Lady's lipstick ended up over most of her face, not just her lips. But her smile was worth it.

Velcro Lady knew the truth. The truth is, it only matters to us where we finish, when we finish, or even *if* we finish. Knowing this liberates those of us in the back of the pack. Knowing this sets us free. We know that by letting go of the illusion of our own importance, we can finally begin to laugh.

On the good days, that realization transfers to the rest of my life and I see that my self-imposed self-importance prevents me from growing. More often than not, it's my imagined fear of what others will think if I fail that keeps me from risking success.

As the number of finish lines that I have crossed accumulates, I begin to understand, too, how important it is to have these opportunities to see a tangible finish to something. So much of our adult lives involves finishing in time frames that our minds can barely comprehend. It's very difficult for me to feel as though I am moving toward the finish line of a thirty-year mortgage or even sixty months of car payments. Those victories, those finish lines, are too distant.

But in a race, even in a marathon, there *is* a finish line. With preparation, courage, persistence, and a little luck, you can cross that finish line. You can take honest pride in having done your best. And for that one moment you can enjoy your achievement.

FINDING SMALL VICTORIES

Before I had real finish lines to cross, I looked for opportunities for small victories to make my life more interesting. Most of these were shallow, of course, like beating someone to a parking space. Others, like getting a two-percent-higher merit pay raise than a colleague, seemed more consequential. Still, they weren't very satisfying.

Running, or more precisely racing, has provided me with finish lines and with opportunities for victories on a regular basis. More important, these personal victories are now measured in minutes and seconds instead of months and years. To finish a 5K in 23:59 is *much* faster than finishing it in 24:01.

I am not alone in this need to finish and the need to feel a sense of victory. Some of the fiercest battles I have ever seen are waged in the middle of the back of the pack by men and women, young and old, who strain against their limitations and push to the edge of their abilities because they must.

I have been engaged in these battles and I can tell you that the competition is as real for 863rd place as it is for 1st. These are pure battles. The reward for winning these personal wars is not prize money or a trophy, or even the recognition of other runners. No, these life-and-death struggles are waged for nothing more than the pleasure of personal satisfaction and the joy of victory.

Sometimes these small victories turn out to be much more significant than we imagine at the time. I was witness to one of these epic battles at a 5K in Nashville, Tennessee. It was the annual Rudolph's Red Nose Run, which attracts over a thousand runners of varying abilities. It is also a costume race, which means you may find yourself challenging Elvis or some other seasonal or cartoon character for position.

I was there with Deborah, a fiftyish friend, who was running her first race. Deborah was new to running and racing, and especially new to the strategies of competition. She lined up near the back of the pack in front of a man wearing a full-sized Styrofoam Gumby costume. It would be easy enough to find victory here, I told her. Just beat Gumby.

But Gumby had other plans. And so began a classic race. Deborah bolted out too fast at the start, then found herself slowing to a walk near the end of the first mile. Sensing her weakness, Gumby began to close. Behind her, Deborah could hear the squeak of Gumby approaching.

She began to run again. Desperately she tried to put some distance between herself and Gumby. The squeak faded. By the turn-around Gumby had fallen behind. Deborah again slowed to a walk, naïvely believing the race was won. But Gumby had saved something. Gumby was trying to run her down! Deborah ran, then walked. Gumby faded, then closed. Back and forth they went for the next mile and a half.

With only a few hundred yards to go, Gumby exploded into a full sprint, like some crazed Styrofoam being. Gumby had a kick! Everyone was screaming—some for Deborah, some for Gumby. Approaching the finish line, they both pushed to their limits. Deborah won. In a time of 36:44.

She had beaten Gumby. Whatever else her life had been or might be, on that day she savored a victory that could never be taken away from her. She had beaten Gumby.

Little did we know at the time how truly significant her victory was. Seven months after beating Gumby, Deborah suffered a severe brain aneurysm. She survived the original episode and the surgery that followed. She fought back to regain some measure of control in her life. She was determined not to lose this battle either.

I like to think that running and racing taught her that she could reach inside of herself for the strength she needed to be victorious. She had discovered the will to win and the desire to finish, and she used those skills to overcome death itself.

LOSING SIGHT OF YOURSELF

Not all finish lines are so important, of course. Most races are just part of the celebration of running. And while it is true that racing can bring out the best in each of us, it can also bring out the worst. The goal to reach the finish line can show us the dignity in our struggle and the struggle of others. If we're not careful, though, it can also bring out the "me as the center of the universe" behavior. I can still get so focused on the finish line that I lose sight of the real message of racing. I lose sight of myself.

I learned this the hard way at a local race. One of the advantages of participating in lots of local races is that you develop a community of racing friends. One of the disadvantages is that the same people beat you race after race. So it was with me and Big Larry.

Compared to my slight stature, Big Larry seems to stand about eight feet tall and to weigh about four hundred pounds. He's not heavy; far from it. He's just big. And strong. It's rumored that he broke the stair climber at our local fitness center.

Big Larry was more than just another racer to me. We worked in the same town and trained at the same health club. We shared stories about our lives. If I needed advice on training or an injury, I often turned to Big Larry. If asked, I'd have said that Big Larry and I were friends.

In the first few years of racing, my main goal was just to keep Big Larry in sight for as long as I could during each event. We raced mostly in 5Ks. If I could still see Big Larry at the end of the first mile, I knew I was having a great race.

I trained hard. Maybe because I was so slow to begin with, there were signs of improvement. In time, I found that I was able to keep Big Larry in sight for more than a mile. In fact, if everything was working, sometimes I actually could see him finish.

That's when it occurred to me—maybe I could beat him! I should have known as soon as the thought entered my head that something was wrong. How could I think of beating him? How could I reduce our friendship to winning and losing? How could I be so consumed with defeating him?

But that fleeting thought became my running mantra. It affected every aspect of my relationship with him. Rather than sharing the joy of his training, I worried that it would make him harder to beat. Rather than celebrating the common ground between us, I allowed myself to believe I had to be better. At every race I lined up thinking, "I can beat him." And at every race, I watched him pull away.

One crisp fall morning, I lined up next to him for a 5K. Still obsessed with beating him, I thought, "This is it. This is the day." "Whadda ya figure to run?" I asked him. "Oh, I'm a little tight. I think I'll just run it," he replied calmly.

What? He was a little tight. Rather than being concerned I thought, "I can do this. I can beat him!" The gun went off, I stayed on his hip, and we ran. At the first mile the volunteer called out the time. "Hey, Larry, we're going out a little fast, aren't we?" I asked. "Uh-huh," was all he said.

So I slowed. But he didn't. I dropped to about ten yards behind him, but couldn't close. I couldn't believe it! He had outsmarted me. I had run the fastest 5K I'd ever run, but I allowed the sweetness of my personal victory to be overcome by my need to beat him.

Another 5K. Another chance. The first half mile was uphill. The wind was in our face. I stayed beside Big Larry rather than letting him block the wind. I wanted to beat him fair and square. At the first mile, the volunteer, again, called out time. It was too fast for an uphill mile into the wind.

He had done it again. He had beaten me in the first mile. Even though I closed in in the final few hundred yards, I never caught him. I was furious. I was angry at him. I was angry at myself. I didn't see what was happening. I didn't see that I was letting something else dictate how I would feel about myself. I didn't see that I was letting racing become another venue for failure.

Then it happened. Big Larry and I were standing yet again at the starting line on an unexpectedly cool summer morning. I was ready to try once more. This time I had a plan. I was not going to go out too fast. I was going to stay inside myself.

I stayed a few yards behind Big Larry for the first two and a half miles. As we rounded the last corner, with less than half a mile to go, I made my move. This is it, I thought. All the training comes down to this. Can I hold this pace for the next few minutes?

Pulling away, I couldn't believe how I felt. I couldn't believe how exciting it was to be in front of Big Larry for the first time. Arms pumping and legs churning, I crossed the finish line, completely spent but satisfied. I had done it.

But my elation was short-lived. I had become so focused on beating Big Larry that I had forgotten that the joy was in the struggle. I had lost sight of the real goal, that of searching for the best inside of me.

And I think I also lost a friend. I turned to find Larry, but he was gone. It has been years now since that race. We've never talked about it. In fact, we haven't raced against each other since. I won that race, but I think I also lost.

Like so many other lessons, I learned this one the hard way. I learned that I am not beyond needing those small victories in my life. I am not beyond risking too much for too little.

I still enjoy racing but something has changed, for the better I think. I still like to challenge myself to do my best, whatever that is on any particular day. But I've come to understand that in doing my best I've got to be careful not to destroy someone else's best effort.

For too long I used the finish line as a measure of my accomplishment. I am more likely now to see the finish line as a threshold, not an obstacle. I am more inclined to view it as a confirmation of my commitment to myself and the sport than as an affirmation of who I am as a runner. I see the clock as a record of the time it took me to run the course, not the value of my effort.

Each race, each finish line, is the end of a chapter in the book that is my life. In some races I exceed my own expectations. Those are chapters with happy endings. In other races, I've seen the finish line from my vantage point inside the straggler's van. Those chapters don't end as happily.

But as I stand at the starting line, I know that somewhere out there is a finish line. And I know that if I only look at what I can do on that day, I will win no matter when, or how, or if, I finish.

12

The Time of Your Life

I like to have a good time. I think most of us do. We spend much of our lives looking for that good time.

As children, especially adolescents, we believe that the good times lie just beyond us. We want time to pass quickly. Getting older is a good thing. But when we are older, we continue to believe we will be able to have a better time at some point in the future than we are having now.

We are sure that those older than us are happier. We are sure that those older than us are enjoying the time of their life. We want to join in the fun. We want the privileges that come with age—driving a car, drinking, voting. As children, and later as adults, we see the passing of time as progress.

It is a sign of advanced age, I suppose, when we begin to think that the best of times are behind us. Unlike children, we believe that those younger than us are the happiest. As we get older we see that the passing of time brings new responsibilities along with the new privileges. We look back and believe that our best times will live only in our memory. It's hard to imagine, as we look in the mirror and see the effects of time on our bodies, that the good times lie ahead of us. We see only the freeze frames of our good times.

For some of us, having a good time became the sole reason to exist. All we wanted was to "let the good times roll." That phrase, in fact, became the mantra of an entire generation. It was impossible to escape the message. In music, in radio and television ads, and on billboards, the message was pervasive. Life was about having good times.

But the good times didn't last. Soon enough, as the children of the sixties shed their tie-dyed shirts and bell-bottom jeans, we discovered that there was never enough time. Time flew, time slipped away. But rarely did time stand still, and it never seemed to roll!

Time eventually became more than the measure of the passing of a day. It became the absolute standard of our productivity and, by extension, of our value. Time couldn't be wasted, because time was money. And time must be well-spent.

Teaching a child to tell time may be a life sentence in anxiety. Before they are taught to tell time, children eat when they're hungry, sleep when they're tired, play when they have the energy, and rest when they're exhausted. How many adults have that wisdom?

Many of us have raised time management to an art form. We have a time for everything, including the time we spend running. We struggle to find time for everything in our lives . . . for everything except the one thing we need most. We never seem to find the time for change.

FINDING THE TIME TO CHANGE

At times I see quite clearly how much running has changed my life. At times I look around me and see all that I have and don't have as a result of my life as a runner. But there was a single moment when I knew that the time had come, when I knew that the change had occurred.

I was attending a professional conference in Chicago. Like at other conferences, the real action was not in the meeting rooms but in the hallways and coffee shops. Careers were made and broken over lunch. Those on the ascendancy tried desperately to be seen in the company of those who had status and prestige.

I had always viewed this particular conference as the most important weekend of my professional life. I planned carefully for weeks in advance to make sure that I would be at the most advantageous spot all the time. I carefully reviewed the meeting topics and breakout sessions and tried to anticipate which would attract the movers and shakers. As in every profession, the high priests and priestesses were to be sought out and honored.

Over the course of the years I had been attending this conference, I had been very successful at placing myself in the presence of the powerful. The decision makers knew my name, knew my face. They knew how eager I was to please, and how ambitious I was to succeed.

But on this morning the whole of my professional life came into sharp focus. The conflict between the person I had been and the person I was becoming reached the boiling point. I stood in my hotel room, dressed in my best professional suit, wearing a well-chosen power tie, prepared to enter this professional Colosseum and meet the lions. I had girded myself well for the battle. I wore my conference badge like a gladiator's shield.

Then I glanced out the window and saw people running along the lakefront path. I was startled. How could this be, I wondered? How could people be free to run mid-morning? Did they not understand that they were missing the opportunity to see and be seen? How could they choose to run?

I stood there for a long minute, looking at the runners. I barely noticed that I was beginning to loosen my tie. Before long I had kicked off my shoes and removed my jacket. Like a person possessed, I threw off my clothes and rummaged for my running shorts.

It was a moment of exhilaration and panic. I had lost control of my senses. What was I doing? What was I thinking? I couldn't do this. Could I? I couldn't actually decide that a run was more important than a professional meeting.

I rode down the elevator in my running shorts, with my colleagues in their best blue blazers and gray slacks. They looked at me like I was crazy. I looked at them and knew that it was they who were crazy. I knew that this was probably the sanest moment of my life.

I realized that where I needed to be at that time was not in a conference seminar or meeting room, but on the paths, running with friends that I didn't know and that I would never meet otherwise. In that instant I saw that I had more in common with those who were running than with those who were not. I finally had found the time to change.

I have never been back to that conference. I have never looked back at what might have been. But I have run those paths along the lake many times since then. Each time I do, I am grateful to those runners who silently beckoned me.

THE SHACKLES OF TIME

I hadn't completely broken free of the shackles of time, though. It was especially true when I entered a race. If I didn't have a good time, I didn't have a good time.

After the first few months of running, the increments of improvement in my race times changed from minutes to seconds. This should come as no surprise. When you start as woefully out of shape as I did, improvement in the early stages is dramatic. With even a little effort, I was able to reduce the time it took me to run a mile.

As I continued to race, however, I realized that although I'd once thought I'd be competitive in no time, it actually would be a long time. Or maybe never. Despite all of the training I was doing, despite all of the time I was spending thinking about running and racing, I wasn't moving up in the pack.

Sometimes I was able to put one or two people between me and the trailing support vehicle. Sometimes I even found myself moving forward, toward the front of the back of the pack. There were even times when I could see the tail end of the back of the middle of the pack.

Then I began to wonder what my hurry was. One time a spectator shouted out in the middle of a particularly miserable race, "And you paid *money* to do this?" After I got over wanting to punch him in the mouth, I began to consider the truth in what he'd asked. Yes, I had paid money. So why was I trying to hurry through the experience?

It occurred to me that if I had paid money to see a movie, I wouldn't want to see it as fast as I could. If I had paid money to take a cruise, I wouldn't want the boat to go as fast as it could. I certainly wouldn't want to go to an amusement park and run from ride to ride at a six-minute pace. Why did I want to hurry through this event?

I know this is contrary to the ethos of the running community. I know it goes against everything that racing supposedly stands for. I know that to be a real racer you should feel like vomiting at the finish line. I know all that, but I don't believe it.

"REAL" MARATHONERS

Like many other revelations, this one came during a marathon. At this marathon, runners who needed more than five hours to finish were allowed to start an hour ahead of the "real" marathoners. I chose the early start. At 7:00 A.M. I found myself running the first mile of my marathon . . . and waving at the busloads of runners, whom I considered to be the real marathoners, who were arriving for the 8:00 A.M. start.

About one thousand of us started early. One thousand runners faced not only the challenge of the distance, but the paralysis of self-doubt. One thousand of us needed to know that we had a cushion, a safety net of time. One thousand of us were willing to identify ourselves as different from the "real" marathoners.

As the miles passed, I drew strength from the runners around me. The "early starters" were a motley collection of people who had trained and were running in the marathon for reasons that escaped most of the real runners. A quiet confidence emanated from this group. These runners had not conceded to their slowness. They had not given in to their lack of speed. On the contrary, in their own way, they all had conquered whatever might have kept them from participating. They had even conquered the community of runners who would never accept them as "real" marathoners.

Near the end of the second hour, the leader went by me. Then the "real" marathoners came past, alone and in groups. Little by little they caught up with us, until we were running with those who hoped to finish in about four hours. Even though I felt more at home with them, they still ran past me.

I had to resist the temptation to run along with them. I had to resist the feeling that because they were running faster, they were running better. I knew that I had found a pace and a rhythm that was working. I knew that I could go no faster, nor slower. And so, one by one, the "real" marathoners passed in and out of my sight, in and out of my life.

Somewhere around mile twenty, it hit me. Instead of a wall, I found the truth. At mile twenty I looked around and saw that not only was I with the "real" marathoners, but I was one of them. I was there. I was doing the miles. I was running at my absolute limit. Just like everyone around me.

I looked at those who, like me, were running in measured strides. I saw the look of determination in their faces. I saw the toll of twenty miles of fighting against an uncooperative body. I saw the strain of overcoming years of failure. I saw it in them, and they saw it in me.

I was a real marathoner. So were they. I was a real runner. So were they. Our slowness is not a measure of our value. Not as individuals, not as runners. We are slow, but we are real.

Sooner or later the running community will recognize that "the times, they are achanging." Today, people who wouldn't have considered becoming runners twenty years ago are coming into the sport of running. As the barriers break down, more and more ordinary people are finding their way into races—from 5Ks to marathons to ultras. Almost to a person, they are in this sport to have a good time.

HAVING THE TIME OF YOUR LIFE

I do not stand in judgment of those who see every race as the moral equivalent of war. There are times when testing my own limits is important. There are times when finding out whether my training is working or whether I can still feel the pleasure that comes from giving a total effort is important, even necessary.

I am saying only that there is another way to look at the time it takes to run a race. Oddly enough and much to my surprise, I began to have better times as I concentrated more on having a good time. As I began to view races as times of celebration, my times actually got faster. Still, in many races, the better the time I was having, the slower my time would be.

Like the Bizarro world of Superman, where everything is back-wards, my idea of a good time seems to be the opposite of everyone else's. When I know early in a race that it just isn't my day, I almost always have a good time. Or so some would say.

On those days I focus on finishing the race in as little time as possible. Those are the days when time passes slowly even though the miles pass quickly. Those are the races that always yield nega-tive splits and PRs in my logbook. But, as Einstein concluded, time is relative.

If it is one of those rare race mornings when everything feels right, if it's one of those days when I line up feeling well-prepared and well-rested, I'll have the best time but have a bad time! On those perfect days, I spend time walking through the water tables, talking to the volunteers. I make sure to take a cup from the youngest child and to high-five every kid along the race route.

On the days when everything's right, I want to take as much time as possible. Those are the days when I'd like to run in a tie-died singlet and bell-bottom running shorts. Those are the times when I really am letting the good times roll. Those are the times of my life!

I hear other runners talk about their glory days. I hear them complain that age has robbed them of speed and stamina. I listen patiently as they tell the stories of races won and nearly won. I try to seem interested as they describe in morbid detail the slow dete-rioration of their bodies.

It's hard for me to understand their concerns. It's hard for me not to think of the time I'm living in right now as my glory years. It's hard for me to imagine a time when I will ever look back and wish I could be like I used to be. I'd rather build my future a minute at a time. I'd rather face whatever is ahead of me when I get there than worry about it now.

I want to take these runners aside and explain to them that, for me, these are the good old days. Somehow, I want them to understand that I am building my future today. My memories are those that I am creating today.

LIVING IN THE MOMENT

Most of us do not have much time on our hands and very few of us have *too* much time on our hands. Those of us who begin running later in life and reach these points of enlightenment well past the midpoint of our lives have precious little time to feel sorry about what we've missed. We are too busy moving forward to spend time looking back.

For us, there is no time to look around for our possibilities. The days of trying to decide what we want to be when we grow up are behind us. We have grown up. At least we've gotten older. Now we have to begin to spend more time accepting what we've become.

Like so much else, you can learn the lesson of "living in the moment" as a runner. You can learn that each step must be taken at its own time and in its own pace. You can learn that it does little good to worry about what you'll do at the finish line until you get there. Every race has to be run one step at a time.

Running teaches us to truly enjoy the moment—to find the happiness that eluded us in the past, the happiness that may not be there in the future—and to concentrate on living in this time of our lives. If we're honest most of us will find, in looking back, that there isn't much to which we want to return. And looking forward is still like staring into the abyss.

Running teaches us that the only time we have is now. The moments that we don't enjoy are lost to us forever. The smile you miss on a young volunteer's face will never be there again. The opportunity to finish someone's first race with them will only happen once.

You must learn to recognize these moments as they are happening, not an hour or a week later.

As you get better at seeing the moment you're in, you'll find that you can stop waiting for the good times to roll. You'll find that you're content to let time march on. And through your running, you will have learned that having the time of your life is often as simple as giving in to the joy of the moment.

Part Four

RUNNING FOR YOUR LIFE

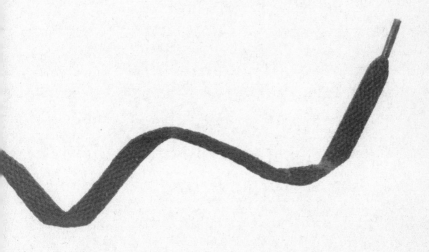

13

Sharing the Joy

Of all the changes that running has brought to my life, the most important one may be the awareness of my need for people. My parents tell the story of when I was a child playing in the sandbox. Other children would come and go, but I was unaffected. I just continued to play.

Many of us learn as children that people will come and go in our lives. We use this as an excuse not to get close to the people around us. As runners, we have the opportunity to break free of our fears of feeling connected. As runners, we can begin to see that, in sharing our effort and in allowing others to share their efforts with us, we can break through the walls of separation.

The ability to continue with or without people in my life carried over into my adulthood. I was casual, even careless, about friendships and relationships. People were interchangeable, even in marriage. I viewed the people around me much like parts on an assembly line. It didn't matter whether they stayed or left; replacements were always available.

I excused myself by rationalizing that this was the result of having spent most of my first forty years as a musician. During that time I became accustomed to spending hours alone in a practice room. I became increasingly comfortable with my own company and increasingly uncomfortable being with anyone else.

For musicians and perhaps others who choose to spend hours

alone, the practice room or office eventually becomes a sanctuary, a safe haven from the pressures of work, relationships, and family. That time alone, even if professionally productive, ultimately leaves many of us unable and unwilling to accept the closeness of another human being. It isn't only musicians who isolate themselves from the world around them. Any profession can become a prison.

When injury ended my career as a performing musician, I found I needed another activity that would require the same kind of discipline, tenacity, and patience. More important, I needed to find an activity that would permit me to spend time by myself. I needed an activity that would sanction my self-containment.

I've met many runners who believe that running will provide that same solitary refuge. They think they will replace the time alone in their personal or professional lives with time alone on the road. They think they will have the same excuse for being antisocial as a runner that I had as a musician. They think they can hide from the responsibilities in their lives by literally running away from them. In time, they discover they are wrong.

I learned the lesson that I need to be with other runners as I have learned so many lessons in my life. I learned it in spite of myself. I didn't go looking for companionship or a place to belong. It was only through the grace and graciousness of more seasoned runners who taught me by their example that I came to see how wrong I was. By embracing me, by welcoming me into their celebration, I came to see the emptiness of my solitary pursuit.

RUNNING WITH OTHERS

The runners who taught me how to share my joy, and theirs, happen to be in the Washington, D.C., area, but there are thousands like them around the country. This motley crew of men and women, academics and government workers, young and not so young, fast and slow, share a weekly ritual of support and affirmation.

Like other running groups, someone among them probably knows how it started, but nobody seems to care at this point. What matters is that this group of runners meets every week, early on Saturday morning, and joins together in celebration of each other and of the community they've created.

It's not that they all actually run together as a group. A few of them do form groups, and as someone takes a few tentative strides down the road or toward the trails, the rest fall into their own comfortable pace, which may range from six-minute miles for the Gazelles to twelve-minute miles for the Penguins like me. The beauty is, it doesn't seem to matter how far or how fast anyone runs.

What does seem to matter is that these runners are together at the start. For a few moments, as the cars pull in and the weary drag themselves out into the morning air, they are a family. The greeting rituals include a handshake or hug and the obligatory, sometimes humorous, review of each other's running attire.

The first time I ran with this group, I was treated like the Prodigal Son, openly welcomed. Absent was the social posturing and strutting that accompanies many gatherings. No one knew or seemed to care about education, income, or any of the other measures we generally use to assess one another. I was wearing running shoes. That was all that mattered.

Now, years later, I have run with hundreds of groups just like this one. I've been welcomed the same way. In every case, it's like discovering that you have friends you've never met.

Of course, many of these weekend runs are only a prelude to the real business of the morning—the post-run meal. Following their runs, the groups invade local eateries, turning them into their clubhouses. The tables get longer and longer as folks finish their runs or bring in their children and spouses. Even those who have "cheesed" by sleeping in instead of running are encouraged to drop by for the breakfast party.

I was always allowed to join the celebration. And I felt a part of the community. With each cup of coffee and each pancake, the walls that usually separated me from the rest of the world began to crumble. In each case, I knew that this was where I belonged.

I began to see that I belong not just with the groups of runners that I have met, but that I belong to an enormous community of runners that I might never meet. There were thousands of other people who were running every day, who were feeling what I was feeling, who thought my goals and dreams were reasonable. It remained only for me to find them.

SEARCHING FOR NEW ROADS AND OLD FRIENDS

One summer I did just that. I went in search of those who would accept me. I left the sandbox, came out of the practice room, and went to find the place where I belong. I went in search of the people who would accept me without question and the community in which I would never have to defend who I was.

The idea was as eloquent as it was simple. It was also as outrageous. My original idea was to stuff a couple of pairs of running shoes and a change of clothes into the saddlebags of a motorcycle, then head across country in search of new roads and new friends.

As with most outrageous ideas, it wasn't long before the idea had transformed itself into a plan. For some reason my good ideas seem to wallow in obscurity in the dark corners of my mind. Outrageous ideas, on the other hand, seem to develop a life of their own. Before I knew it, the motorcycle was packed and I was on the road.

The plan was to ride cross country, from Nashville to Washington, D.C., to Portland and San Diego, then back. Eight weeks of riding and running and racing. Eight weeks without the tools and trappings of adulthood—no garage-door opener, no microwave, no closet full of clothing and shoe choices. On a motorcycle, if you can't stuff it, you can't take it.

As the departure date approached and the unthinkable became inevitable, what came into clear focus was how running has changed my life. This trip, this concession to my chronic wander-lust, was not a journey away from it all, as other trips had been. It was different. It was not a trip of soul searching and introspection. This was a journey of celebration.

The purpose of the journey, if it needed a purpose, was to run new roads and meet old friends. The odd part was that some of those old friends were people I'd never met. Yet, time after time, as I described the metamorphosis that running had produced in my life, I found that it was identical to someone else's.

At every stop, I found people who shared my love of running, my struggle to move past my self-imposed limitations, and my determination to overcome an earlier life of poor decisions, bad judgment, and abject ignorance. I ran with new and veteran runners and discovered how little difference there was among us.

At the beginning of the trip I believed my story was somehow unique. By the end I knew I was just one of many people—young and old, male and female—who had found themselves through running. By the time the trip was over, a most remarkable transition had occurred. The solitude I expected to feel was replaced by a sense of belonging. Rather than feeling isolated in my odyssey, I was buoyed by the knowledge that others had gone before me and had been successful, and that still others were behind me on the same path.

For fifty-six days in twenty-one states, I was among friends. On mornings when I ran by myself I knew that I wasn't running alone. I saw other runners and knew that we had something in common. I waved, smiled, and felt welcomed.

FINDING THE JOY AT HOME

As wonderful as it was to feel this bond with friends, the most remarkable change of sharing the joy of running occurred right at home. The greatest joy was to discover that my wife, and friend, was also the best running partner anyone could ever have.

Karen started running several months after I did. I suppose that she, like me, was waiting for this latest obsession to fade. I didn't blame her for waiting. In the years we had been married she had watched patiently as dream after dream went up in smoke. She had watched me pursue each new activity with passion, only to have the passion die when failure became inevitable.

In the early stages, when we ran together, I made the "manly'" gesture of running slowly, to stay with her. Not wanting to discourage her, I ran back and forth, even backwards, in a convoluted attempt to be supportive. In spite of me, she continued to run.

As the weeks and months passed and as Karen's skill and ability became more obvious, it became harder and harder for me to maintain the charade that I was holding back. Day by day, like magic, she was becoming a runner.

We began racing nearly every weekend and Karen began winning age-group awards nearly every weekend. We joked that she was trophy sniffing at every race and that she would pout if she didn't come away with hardware.

I consoled myself by reminding myself that winning age-group awards in the forty-plus women's age groups was easier because fewer women were entered. It was true, but it also allowed me to miss the point that Karen was becoming a very good runner. This formerly quiet and soft-spoken librarian was becoming a strong, lean, running machine.

She raced at every distance, and she took home awards at nearly every distance. Little by little our back room began to look like a warehouse. The shelves filled with trophies and ribbons and plaques, evidence of the change that was taking place in her life, and in mine, although I didn't realize it at the time.

We ran her first marathon together, a cold, miserable affair that we easily could have quit. Mile after mile I waited for her to give up. Mile after mile she hunkered down. She was determined to finish, and she did.

Then she set her sights on qualifying for the hundredth running of the Boston Marathon. That decision set in motion a chain of events that changed our lives forever. Each mile of training brought us closer and closer to the most important moment of our lives together.

In every relationship, events occur that change the very fabric of the relationship. Some of these are obvious: the birth of a child, the death of a loved one. We can prepare for some of these events, while others catch us completely off guard.

IT ALL COMES DOWN TO A SINGLE STEP

I never expected that one of those moments would occur at mile twelve of a marathon. That would have been my last guess. But one did occur for me, in the middle of nowhere and without warning, at the twelfth mile of the Fox Cities Marathon.

It's amazing, really. Amazing how months of planning, miles and miles of training can all come down to one step. More amazing in this case is how the years of being in a relationship can be crystallized into a single moment, a single step.

The day began innocently enough. Karen was trying to qualify for Boston. Oh, sure, she'd only been running for three years and her only previous marathon was a walk/run/shuffle/drag affair that lasted over five hours, but Boston was her dream.

More important, in the fifteen years that we had been married, it was the first dream that was really, truly hers. It was the first time we had organized our lives around who she wanted to be, rather than who I wanted to be. It was the first time she had asked as much of me as I had asked of her.

We had run hundreds of miles together in preparation for the marathon: long slow runs, tempo runs, speed work. We ran them all side by side and stride for stride—until we gradually began to run as a unit. Everyone thought I was pacing her. But down deep, I knew the truth. I was hanging on for dear life.

As the weeks wore on and the training grew more intense, the differences between us became more obvious. My body—a body that had endured too much booze, too many cigarettes, and too many late nights—was reaching its limits. As the mileage increased, so did the reality of my ability.

But Karen's body welcomed the challenge and the miles. Slowly, her legs became the legs of a runner—a *real* runner, with strength and stamina and style. I watched in stunned disbelief as her shape became that of a trim and youthful athlete.

The plan was simple enough. Run the marathon together, as we had trained for it. Run as one, side by side. But life had an altogether different plan.

The early miles of the race passed perfectly. Striding together, in sync, we chatted and laughed as we ran. But, little by little, the demons in my left knee made their presence known. Little by little, the knee began to tighten. I knew it was only a matter of time.

At mile twelve, it happened. One step, a sinister snap, and it was over. The marathon plan, and the relationship as it had been, ended in that instant. With that one single step, everything changed, and I knew that my life, *our* life, could not, would not, ever be the same again.

I pulled up; I had no choice. But Karen did. Her choice was to choose between her dream and my reality, between what she knew was best for her and what she thought was best for me. At that moment, she had to confront her own strength in the face of my weakness.

As I watched her continue to run, as she slowly but surely moved gracefully away, toward her dream, I knew that this was a moment of truth. We were letting go. Letting go of each other. Letting go of ourselves. We were each facing the truth about ourselves. We were each facing the truth about the other.

The seemingly innocent dishonesty that inevitably creeps into a relationship became suddenly and vividly obvious. I was not always to be strong. She was not always to be caring. She could accomplish something that would elude me. She could be better than me. We were letting go of the illusion of equality and grasping for the first time the truth of being separate and alone—but still in love.

Running brought us both to ourselves, and to each other. Running allowed us both to be who we are and taught us to find joy in each other. More than anything else, it has shown us how to be: how to be together, how to be apart, how to be a couple, and how to be individuals.

Karen didn't qualify for the hundredth Boston Marathon that day. She tried again later that same year and missed qualifying by a matter of minutes. In a funny twist of fate, two days after her second attempt, my name was drawn in the lottery to run the hundredth. And as luck or destiny would have it, Karen found a way to run it with me. Together we celebrated the goal that had brought us to ourselves.

BEING PART OF A COMMUNITY OF RUNNERS

There are still times when I prefer to run alone, when the rhythmic pounding of my shoes against the pavement is the only thing that brings me the solace I need. There are times when the miles are the only protection I have against the demons.

But I know now that there are also days when it isn't the miles but the people who are the most important part of the training. There are times when sharing the joy of running, with a single individual or a group, is necessary to complete myself.

Those are the days when pushing my fear of being close to another human being does me more good than pushing my heart rate. Those are the days when finding the right words is much more difficult than finding the right pace.

Too often we run only within the confines of our own world. We believe that the joy of solitude is enough. We believe that it is only during the times when we run alone that we can find the answers to life's questions. We have favorite routes and favorite races. And if we don't run alone, we run always with the same group or partner.

If we stay in our own world too long, though, we can easily come to believe that the universe of running is the world within our reach. It isn't true. Our universe is as big, or as small, as we make it.

The joy we feel in running multiplies as we share it with others. When we break free of our own goals and see how we can contribute to someone else's goals we take running to another level. Running becomes not only a solitary activity, to be pursued alone, but a conduit through which we can connect to those closest to us, even to those unknown to us.

On your next run, throw your shoes in a bag and head out of town. If you're a city runner, drive to the country. If you run in the country, try downtown. Cross a county line. Go over a state border. Call a friend. Walk with him. Talk with him. Help him discover the joy in running. Help him understand the joy in finding yourself. Help him realize there is more to running, and more to you, than miles run. Discover for yourself that you are part of a community of runners.

Once you begin to share the joy, once you begin to seek out those who are willing to share their joy with you, you may find, as I did, the truth in the words of Robert Earl Keen, Jr.: "The road does go on forever, and the party never ends."

14

The Warrior Penguin

It happens every time we pin on a race number. Somehow, the act of attaching the number to the front of our shirt begins the metamorphosis. As we ceremoniously thread the safety pin through one of the holes on the four corners of our race number and watch the pin disappear beneath the fabric, as we cautiously avoid pinning the number directly to our skin, we are transformed.

Moments before, we were mere mortals. Now, standing proudly in front of the mirror, checking to see that the number is straight and properly placed, we are warriors. In that instant, like all great warriors, our lives are reduced to the battle before us. Like all great warriors, we stand ready to face the enemy. In most cases, that enemy is ourselves.

I doubt that the Roman legions had exactly the same look. Our battle regalia, after all, includes double-layer socks, CoolMax T-shirts, and mesh-sided running caps. I doubt that ancient warriors tied and retied their boots twenty-seven times or used little plastic "squeezies." Nonetheless, this ritual of girding ourselves with sunscreen and Runner's Lube, of arming ourselves with packets of energy gel, and finally strapping on our water carrier and holstering the bottle, is just as important to us as the battle rituals of the Roman legions were to them.

Once everything is in place, we make our way to the tracks and roads and cities and parks. We go in search of others who are prepared to face the challenge of the course, the challenge of the competitors around us, and, most important, the challenge of our own expectations.

The search begins at the starting line. Person by person, we move among the assembled warriors to find those with whom we can share this moment. For me, this means moving toward the *back* of the assembled runners. But on my way toward the back, I absorb energy from each person I pass. The nervousness, the joking, the pacing, are all part of the pre-battle scene. Finally, when I have reached the back, I have found my company of warriors.

We runners in the rear echelon, in the Penguin Brigade as I call it, are an odd assortment of shapes, sizes, ages, and genders. The back of the pack is the ultimate melting pot. There are always some in the back who are entering their first battle. The veterans gather around, giving them support and advice. There are always some, too, who are more accustomed to being close to the front. Injury or illness has brought them to us during this battle. We welcome them, although all of us in the back are aware that once they have recovered, they will make their way back up to their former ranks.

At the command of start, at the sound of the gun or cannon, we stand ready. We "stand" ready because after those in the front start running, there is almost always a delay before we in the rear can begin to move forward. Eventually, standing evolves into running in place which evolves into walking. Finally, as we approach the starting line, the rear guard begins to run.

FACING THE ENEMY WITHIN

*T*hat is when the real battle begins. Our battles are not for position or for awards. Our battles are most often not even with one another.

All of us have come to this place and donned our armor to face our most brutal enemy—ourselves.

We are battling our fears and insecurities. We are battling our history. We are slaying the dragons of our past failures. For each of us, it is a battle to the death. There can be no negotiated peace in this battle. It is the battle of, and for, our lives.

I was witness to this collective battle one year at the Marine Corps Marathon, in Washington, D.C. I watched as the runners gathered in the pre-race dawn. Alone and in groups, they made their way to the starting line. Some chatted, while others paced silently, lost in their thoughts and fears. As we waited, as the count-down to the battle commenced, I listened to the conversations around me.

The more outspoken of the veterans shared their insights on the physical and emotional toll exacted by running 26.2 miles. They did not try to frighten their fellow runners. They only tried to help them prepare for the battle ahead. The advice ranged from the practical to the prophetic.

At the appointed time, the cannon fired. Slowly, tentatively, but defiantly we began. Together, but alone, we chased our dreams and our demons. Some faced the marathon challenge for the first time. Others were there to prove that they could still overcome the distance. Whatever their reasons, whatever their strategy, the waiting was over. The battle had begun.

On that particular day, the challenge for me was to finish intact and unhurt. It had been two years since I had completed a marathon on my own terms. Two years of conceding that the strength of my will could not overcome the weakness of my body. Two years of hitting walls, breaking down, and limping in.

Over five hours later, charging up the final hill to the Iwo Jima monument, with a fellow warrior and first-time marathoner, to the cheers of the crowd and the encouragement of the Marines, I knew we both had won our battles that day.

PLAYING HURT

Not all battles are victories, and not all victories are so sweet. There are times when, like all warriors, one must decide that discretion is the better part of valor. There are times when winning the war means losing the battle. And there are times when the real battle is with the fear of what it means not to finish.

There is no shame in deciding that finishing a race is not worth the risk. There are times when what's best for your running and racing is to stop. Such times may result from injury or sickness, or they may result from a plain lack of desire. Every experienced runner will acknowledge that there are days when racing well means not racing at all. There are times when the risk of competing is not worth the risk of injury or burnout. There are times when even the most devoted warrior must sit out the battle.

This is a difficult lesson to learn. Many of us are so accustomed to thinking of ourselves as quitters that we go too far to the other extreme and believe that we must persevere at any cost. If we are not careful we can forget that there are times when quitting, in a race or in training, will allow us eventually to continue the battle.

For many of us, the battle with being a quitter starts with turning a deaf ear to the fatigue or pain in our bodies. Ignoring your body is a dangerous game and one that you will ultimately lose. There is nothing heroic about running and racing through injury and pain. It is not a sign of courage that you can push your threshold of pain to higher and higher levels. Ignoring your body is often a sign that the real enemy is still the demon living inside your soul.

Many adult-onset athletes turn to running as a release from self-destructive behaviors like drinking, smoking, or drugs. Many shift the obsessiveness that led to such abusive behavior into their new lives as runners. They replace one addiction with another that is more socially acceptable.

But an irrational and self-destructive addiction to running is no healthier than many other addictions. Being unable to decide when you should stop or reduce your running because it's healthier physically or emotionally to do so is a sure sign that the issues that drove you to your previous addictive behavior are still alive and well in your psyche.

Make no mistake, I am not immune to such forms of Russian roulette. I have taped, wrapped, and medicated myself on far too many occasions in foolish attempts to squeeze just one more mile or one more race out of a muscle or joint. I speak not out of a sense of judgment but as one who is struggling to reform himself.

When I started running, I was convinced my transformation from unhealthy to healthy behavior was complete and absolute. I was sure that because I no longer reached for a cigarette or a drink when I was stressed or down or unhappy, I had made peace with all my demons. It wasn't true.

I was startled to learn that as a runner I was still capable of treating my body as an entity that was separate from me. Even as a runner I believed that when I abused my body, it would forgive me. Even as a runner, I didn't see that I could still damage my body.

Eventually I learned that being a warrior means being strong enough to decide which battles you will fight and which you will walk away from. Being a warrior means knowing your heart and soul, as well as your body. Being a warrior means not only knowing what you are fighting for, but whom you are fighting against. For many of us, the greatest battle is within ourselves.

More surprising than discovering the warrior within us when we pin on our race numbers is discovering that the warrior spirit is there even when we are not racing. As we dig deeper to find the courage to battle new courses and new distances, we discover that we can find that courage whenever we need it.

Our confidence in what we are and who we are grows as we win more victories over ourselves. As we face the worst in ourselves, we also have to confront the best in ourselves. One race and one day at a time, we can create a new myth for ourselves. One step at a time, we write our own legends.

Many people spend their entire lives desperately trying to avoid that moment of truth when they will have to face honestly who they are, who they have been, and what they may become. They hide behind a self-created façade of wealth, intellect, or even success. They may convince themselves that the image is intended for others, but very often the person they most want to hide from is themselves.

As runners, we cannot hide from the moments of truth when we must look at ourselves honestly. Instead, we must actively seek out opportunities to face ourselves, to challenge ourselves, to take stock of ourselves, and to move past the lies we used to tell ourselves. Rather than seeking shelter from the truth, we are compelled to stand firm and weather the storm of enlightenment and self-discovery.

THE FACES OF FAILURE

These moments of enlightenment can come at the most unlikely times—when we least expect them and when we are least able to accept them. As runners and warriors, we must always be prepared to face these emerging revelations when they are presented to us.

There have been many such revelations for me, but none so profound as the one I faced on a deserted stretch of highway outside of Muncie, Indiana. I remember that moment of enlightenment as if it happened yesterday, and the very thought causes the hair on my arms to stand up.

The occasion was a half Ironman-distance triathlon called the Muncie Endurathon. The event consisted of a mile and a quarter swim, a fifty-six-mile bicycle ride, followed by a half-marathon (13.1 mile) run. I had never attempted anything of this magnitude

before. Although I felt prepared for the event, I wasn't at all prepared for what would happen.

The swim and the bike ride were relatively uneventful. I was
nearly last out of the water, and by the end of my bike segment, many
of the leaders had finished their race. By the time I started the run,
the temperature, which had climbed all day, was well into the 90s.

The run was an out-and-back course through unshaded Indiana
cornfields. As I racked my bike to begin the half-marathon, I could
see faster competitors finishing the event. As I began running, I
also could see still others walking and staggering through the latter miles of the half-marathon. I thought of the four hours of effort
behind me and the three hours or more that stretched ahead of me,
taking little comfort in seeing those who were so much stronger
than me giving in to the ravages of the course and the day.

As I settled into a pattern of running when I could and walking
when I couldn't, it was clear that this was becoming a battle not
just with my tiring body, but with my increasingly weary spirit.
Time and again I reached down to find something extra in my soul.
Time and again it was there.

Then, at about mile eleven, it happened. I saw a vision—a wall,
really, of faces. There, in front of me, were the assembled images of
all the people who had ever called me a failure. They were as real as
if they had been standing directly in my way.

They were all there. The elementary-school teachers who misunderstood dyslexia and labeled me forever as an underachiever.
The physical education teachers and coaches who ridiculed my less
well-developed physical stature. They were all there. The faces of
failed relationships and failed friendships.

The entire cast of every failure in my past came to life on that
road in Indiana. They had gathered to see me fail once again. I
could hear them telling me that there was no shame in giving up.
Why should this day be any different? I could just sit down beside
them. I could quit. I could stop running. I was tired. I was hot. I
was tempted.

Then something truly remarkable happened. As if possessed, I found myself actually picking up my pace. In stark defiance of this chorus of the voices of defeat, I chose to continue. I ran through them. I ran right through the wall of my own memory.

I ran for the next two miles. I ran mostly because I was afraid— afraid that the faces of failure would catch me, afraid that they would reassemble in front of me again. And afraid that this time I wouldn't have the strength or the courage to run through them.

Seven and a half hours after I started, I finished. I crossed the finish line, sat down, and began to sob. It was not an ordinary cry of relief, or sorrow, or even joy. This pain was not coming from my body. These tears were not just from this day. These were tears born of a lifetime of failing.

I cried for the six-year-old who couldn't run as fast as the others. I cried for the twelve-year-old who couldn't hit the ball or catch like the others. I cried for all the times I stood alone, waiting to be chosen. I cried for the teenager who knew nothing about life and for the young man who knew nothing about love.

My wife came to meet me and I looked up and said to her: "It's such a long way. Such a long, long way." I'm sure she thought I meant the course. I didn't. I meant that it is such a long way for many of us to travel before we find ourselves.

FINDING THE WARRIOR

I found the warrior in me that day. At mile eleven I dug deep enough to find the courage that was buried under years of self-imposed cowardice. I faced my memories of all those who had convinced me that I would fail, and of all those who would have me continue to fail. I met the enemy, and it was me.

We can't pin race numbers on our shirts all day every day, but I wish we could. I wish we could stand in front of the rude salesperson or angry co-worker with a race number pinned to our chests. I wish we could wear that outward reminder of the warrior in us. Not so much for them as for ourselves.

That race number can remind us that we've looked carefully at ourselves and have defined ourselves in our own terms. It can remind us that we have weaknesses, but also that we have strengths. It can remind us of what we can and cannot do, of what we are and what we are not. It can remind us that the victory is in knowing the truth.

In the end, there is a calmness in being a runner and a warrior. There is a quiet confidence that comes from knowing you have survived the heat of the race and the battle. There is a poise that comes from knowing the depths of your own resolve.

There may be other ways to find that calm, but for many of us, nothing works as well as running. Standing at the starting line, knowing that we have trained and sacrificed to take on the challenge, fills us with a self-assurance that nothing else can.

In surviving the heat of the battle, we come to understand that the victory of each run, the victory of each race, has nothing to do with winning or losing. It has nothing to do with finishing a run or a race that truly shouldn't be finished. It has to do with learning how to be who you honestly are, at every moment.

15

Failing to Fail

All of us want to be successful, but most of us have our own definitions of success. For some, success is a beautiful house or a fast car. Others define success in terms of money earned or money saved. Whatever our definition of success may be, very few of us want to be failures.

Yet success itself, or more likely the external manifestation of success, often becomes our goal. Getting the house, the car, or the money becomes the driving force in our lives. And then success has a way of regenerating itself into more success—into bigger houses, faster cars, and even more money. Nothing succeeds like success, as the saying goes, but it can become a vicious cycle that controls our lives.

Even if we achieve these external measures of success, deep in our psyche many of us believe that we have been truly successful at only one thing in our lives. We believe that we have only been successful at failing. In fact, if we are not careful, we become so successful at failure that our lives are dedicated to finding more and more successful ways to fail.

We take on projects or jobs that we are doomed to fail at in order to bolster our negative view of ourselves. We undermine relationships and sabotage friendships. If nothing else works, we destroy— by malicious neglect—anything that might keep us from succeeding at failing.

This may sound contradictory, but it isn't. Succeeding feels good. We all like to feel good. And success is reinforcing. It makes us feel more and more sure of ourselves. If we are successful at failing, we reinforce the notion that we are failures and become more and more convinced that it is true.

Unfortunately, we live in a culture that provides us with a multitude of opportunities to succeed at failure. Every day we are able to find other people who have more (or less) of whatever it is we use to measure success. Every day we can congratulate ourselves for seeking out new confirmation of our success at failing.

Of all the ways to succeed at failing, none has had a more profound impact on the American population's psyche than the diet and fitness industries. The success of these industries relies on failure. For them to be successful, we must fail. They must make *sure* that we fail. If we, the dollar-spending consumers, succeeded at dieting and getting into shape, the diet and fitness industries would disappear within a year.

They prey not only on our need to fail, but also on our seemingly endless ability to believe the unbelievable. When we hear about a new diet program or fitness machine, we suspend all rational thought. When every fiber of our body and soul knows that there is *no way* we ever will look like the person selling us the machine or diet, we want to believe. And we do. We believe even though we know the end result will be failure.

Unless you have been living on a different planet for the past fifty years, you know that diets don't work. Machines that move, shake, or twist you don't work. You cannot look like a supermodel by using anything for five minutes a day, three days a week. We all know that. So why do people insist on trying one fad diet or magic machine after another? To succeed at failing. It is so important to succeed that we will do almost anything to avoid failing at failure.

By the time we reach adulthood most of us are so adept at failing that we no longer fear it. Failing comes naturally. It requires almost no effort. When you fail, your world, your view of yourself, and everything around you stay the same. There's no risk! If, on the other hand, you succeed, everything changes. Most of us are not afraid to fail. We are afraid to succeed.

IT'S OKAY TO FAIL

*B*ut it's okay to fail! Better still, you can fail to be a failure. How? By learning a new definition for success. You can start by accepting that the biggest risk for you is not the risk of failing. It is the risk of succeeding.

When I am honest with myself I must admit that there have been many times in my life when I have chosen the security of failure over the unexplored waters of success. I have often snatched defeat from the jaws of victory. I have stood on the threshold of certain success, then turned and walked away. If you're honest with yourself, you have, too.

Part of the problem is that success is not static. Success is not an absolute goal that, once achieved, satisfies one's need to succeed forever. There are always higher mountains to climb. Success is a moving target and an evasive one at that. But the very elusive nature of success is the key to understanding how to achieve both immediate and long-term success. By understanding success, we can avoid the vortex of failure into which we so often fall.

Too many individuals find themselves in diet and fitness programs that are doomed from the beginning because the goal, the definition of success, is too rigid. The books and charts and graphs are designed for the average person. But none of us is average. Each of us is unique. Any program that locks us into prescribed goals ultimately will not work.

It is not only people who are new to running, or health and fitness, who are tempted to look to objective models for success. Even among highly trained athletes, the notion of absolute goals often leads to frustration and wanting to quit. It doesn't matter if success is defined as losing ten pounds in one month or qualifying for the Boston Marathon, rigid and inflexible goals are a formula for failure.

FLEXIBLE DEFINITIONS OF SUCCESS

At 26.2 miles, the marathon, more than any other running event, serves as the best example of the necessity for a flexible definition of success. When I first contemplated training to run a marathon, I thought my goal would be to complete 26.2 miles. Some runners may train to complete the distance within a certain time, but I wanted only to finish on the same day that I started.

As I began to prepare, as I began to focus more clearly on the goal of finishing, the risk of injury quickly became very real. Whether one is preparing for a three- or a five-hour marathon, the injury rate skyrockets as the miles of training begin to accumulate. As nagging pain began to affect my training, finishing was no longer the goal. I redefined success as figuring out a way to *begin* the marathon in good health.

If everything works and you are fortunate enough to get to the starting line of the marathon, your goal on race morning may indeed be to finish the 26.2 miles. At the start you may be looking at the entire marathon, the total mileage and total time, as the only unit of success. I discovered, though, that the ability to remain flexible in defining success *during* the marathon ultimately was the deciding factor in whether I would succeed or fail. I quickly dismissed the idea of completing 26.2 miles as my sole definition of success. I understood that success in the marathon was not a matter of running 26.2 miles. No, success in a marathon is running one step at a time, and doing that for 26.2 miles.

Most experienced marathoners will tell you that the halfway point in a marathon is not, as one might think, 13.1 miles. Almost all runners will tell you that the halfway point is mile twenty. Many, myself included, are convinced that there are usually eight and a half miles between mile markers twenty-two and twenty-three.

The physical, mental, and emotional toll extracted by the final 6.2 miles of the marathon is enormous. In those final miles, my definition of success changed minute by minute. Completing 26.2 miles was a forgotten concept. Seeing each new mile marker was cause for celebration, and completing one more mile became my new definition of success. Eventually, success came down to running one more step. Picking my foot up and putting it down just one more time became my working definition of success.

In the end, becoming a successful marathoner meant taking just one step. Success became a matter of stepping across the finish line. With that single step, I succeeded. With that single step, and all the other single steps that preceded it, I became successful.

As important as that final step was, it was no more important than every step that came before it. It is easy to believe that it was the final step alone that made me successful, but my success was really the result of thousands of steps that had come before. It was hundreds of miles of preparation and training, days and weeks of planning that got me successfully to the finish line. Not just that last step.

The day of my first marathon, I learned to allow my definition of success to change. I learned that I am not always capable of conceptualizing giant, long-range plans for success in my head. I learned that, for me, success would have to occur in increments small enough and flexible enough to grasp. My success would come one step at a time.

I began setting goals in my running and weight-control program that were just as fluid. Whether my long-range goal was to lose ten pounds or one hundred pounds, I had to break it down into achievable but flexible increments. As with the marathon, I had to take many small steps if I wanted to reach the finish line.

Success became the accomplishment of hundreds of intermediate steps rather than achieving a single, grandiose goal. My success at weight control became the healthy choice of food in front of me at a particular moment. I didn't have to control what I ate for the rest of my life; I only had to control what I was eating right now.

The ability to constantly redefine success is one of the surest means of becoming successful. Success is a habit. So is failing. A dynamic definition of success, one that takes into account the reality of the moment, is far more effective in establishing the habit of succeeding than is an inflexible definition.

I wanted to be a successful runner. The more I ran, the more I knew that running was going to be more than a sport to me. It was going to be more than just an activity. Running was going to be my way to learn to fail at failure.

RUNNER'S BLOCK

*E*ven though I wanted to run for the rest of my life, I couldn't imagine being a runner for the rest of my life. I couldn't imagine that I would ever become anything other than a person who ran. At first I thought that the only time I was a runner was when I was running. But, as with so many other things, I was wrong. I had to find the place in my soul where I would become a runner. To be a runner, I had to learn what it meant to *fail* as a runner.

This is not as confusing as it sounds. It's a matter of accepting all of what it means to be a runner. It means not only accepting the parts of running that bring satisfaction, but embracing the times when running is frustrating or boring or both. It means accepting that not wanting to run is as much a part of running as wanting to run.

The truth is, whether you've been running for a month or a lifetime, there are days when you don't want to run. There are days when running just doesn't work. There are days when to be successful, you must fail to run. I call it runner's block.

Runner's block doesn't happen to me on days when I shouldn't run, of course. Oh, no. For some reason, on the days when I've got a little ache or a new pain or am feeling extra stiff, I can't wait to run. On those days I am like a tight pair of pants, ready to rip. On those days, I have to tie myself to a chair to avoid turning a minor inconvenience into a full-blown crisis.

No, for some reason runner's block affects me most on the days when I feel great, when the weather is perfect, when I have plenty of time, and yet I simply don't want to run. For me, it is sometimes the days when running should be the easiest that it's the most difficult.

Like the first signs of coming down with a cold, I can tell the symptoms of an impending case of runner's block. I know I'm having an attack when I sit down for a minute to change clothes and find myself so interested in a rerun of *Gilligan's Island* that I don't move for thirty minutes. When I get so wrapped up in whether the good professor's new contraption will really save castaways, I know that my runner's block is at fever pitch.

I used to try to fight it. I went through the motions of getting ready for a run. I picked out a pair of shoes, then found myself just staring at them. Sometimes I set out a pair of shorts and a shirt, then walked away.

Other times I actually got dressed, walked out the door, started down the driveway, and then turned around. The farthest I ever got was about half a block from the house. I started my watch, began running, stopped the watch, turned around, and walked home.

I used to worry about what it meant when I didn't want to run. I thought that runners always wanted to run. I thought that failing to run was failing as a runner. I was afraid that if I missed a day or two, I wouldn't be a runner anymore.

Then I began to understand that it isn't my body that wants to run every day—it's my head. There are times when my legs know they have plenty of mileage for the week, but my head keeps thinking about the logbook. How will the graph look if I don't get in those extra three miles?

I worried, too, about the mileage bragging sessions. When I was involved in motor sports, everyone bragged about horsepower. With runners, it's mileage. What will I say when someone asks me how many miles I got in this week? I've decided it's best to handle mileage the same way I used to handle horsepower. Lie about it.

Some days it's still a matter of just getting started. Those are the days when I tell myself that as long as I'm dressed, I might as well run a little. On those days, once I'm started and feeling good about running, I just keep going.

When runner's block hits me, it is like a kind of paralysis. It stops me dead in my tracks. I can't will myself through it, I can't force myself through it, and I certainly can't *run* though it. I just have to wait it out. I have to allow myself to fail to run in order to succeed at being a runner.

Fortunately, runner's block doesn't affect me very often. Most days, the time I spend running is the most important time of the day. It's often what happens during my run that makes what happens during the rest of the day tolerable.

Now I understand the importance of failing to run. As important as discipline and consistency are in a lifelong running program, for me nothing is as unpleasant or unproductive as making myself run. I finally figured out how important running was to me. Now, on those few days a year when I just don't want to run, I just don't. On those days, I fail to fail.

UNDEFEATED SEASONS

I suppose if I ever had a perfect year, a year with no frustrations and no failures, I'd give up running. If I ever had a year when everything went right, when every training run was purposeful and every race was a PR, I'd be inclined to quit.

As a matter of fact, I had a year like that—my very first year as a runner. That year I was well organized. I trained according to a plan. I raced according to a schedule. And I PR'd at every distance I ran. What a wonderful year! I was undefeated. Oh, I failed to win every time I raced. Sometimes I was beaten by everyone else in the race. But I was never defeated.

That year I ran my first 5K. I had trained hard. I was sure I could run the distance. What I didn't expect was the intensity of effort. I was surprised by my reaction to competition during the race. I didn't know how much I would want to pass other runners and how much I would *not* like being passed.

Early in that first season I confused not winning with losing. I believed the T-shirt that said "Second place is the first loser." I believed that runners who didn't win had failed. During that time, as I sat dejectedly through the award ceremonies, I thought the only winners were the runners who were getting trophies.

I hadn't yet grasped the dignity of those who run without hope of victory but are far from hopeless runners. I had yet to understand the difference between success and failure. I had yet to understand that I could never fail if my effort was real. I had yet to understand that, indeed, for many runners, the miracle isn't that they finish, but that they have the courage to start.

That first year I set distance goals: 10K, 15K, and a half-marathon. With each completed race, I felt a curious mix of satisfaction and confusion. I was satisfied that I had finished but confused that I wasn't moving toward the front of the pack. I wasn't failing, but it didn't feel exactly like success either.

Relying on the Type A personality that had become my nature, and not knowing any better, I trained more and raced harder, farther and more often. I was so intent on not failing that every starting line became the moral equivalent of war.

Getting an age-group award became my private search for the Holy Grail. But age-group awards weren't forthcoming. In large races I sometimes made it into the upper half. In smaller, local races, I often was last in my age group. For the life of me, I didn't know why.

Lacking fundamental good sense, at the end of my first year of running I decided to run a marathon. Looking back, I'm sure that the unspoken plan was to fail, and in failing, to give myself the chance to quit running, to quit losing, to quit having to redefine my idea of success.

It almost worked. By December of that first year, I was so overtrained even my hair hurt. A week before the marathon, I started my taper. For seven days, I did absolutely nothing. For seven days, my muscles tightened and my joints swelled.

My appointment with failure came on a cold, damp morning in Memphis, Tennessee. The freezing temperature and light rain sealed my fate. What had begun with the promise of success ended just minutes later in abject failure.

I didn't make it to the first mile marker before my body began to lock up. I didn't get to the first of the twenty-six mile markers before my knees and hips deserted me. That was it! My race was over. It was the worst I had ever failed. It wasn't just that I was the last runner to finish. This time I was the first to quit. Had I failed? Yes. Was I a failure? No!

I knew that if I still wanted to be a runner after that day, I would always want to be a runner. If a one-mile marathon didn't send me back to a life of overindulgence and inactivity, nothing would. If I failed to fail *that* day, then every other day would be successful.

Since that inauspicious beginning, I have run many other marathons. From that moment of failure came the strength and wisdom that led to success. From that failure, I learned what real success means. Real success is failing to fail. Real success is looking honestly at what you can do, and then setting out to do more. Real success is knowing that failure is nothing more than a component of success.

16

Running for Your Life

There are a hundred good reasons to start running. Running promotes cardiovascular fitness. It may lower your blood pressure. It may help you to lose or control your weight. The list goes on. There are also hundreds of bad reasons to start running. Among them is that running promotes cardiovascular fitness. It may lower your blood pressure. It may help you to lose or control your weight, etc.

For all the good and bad reasons to start running, most runners find that there is only one reason to keep running. In order to run for your life, running has got to be fun. It may do all sorts of wonderful things to your heart and lungs, but in the end, none of that will matter if it's not fun.

Keeping your running fun shouldn't be all that difficult, yet it seems to be one of the biggest obstacles for new runners. Some of the reasons are trying to run too far or too fast, or trying to live up to your own, or someone else's, unrealistic expectations. But those reasons alone don't explain why running isn't fun for some runners.

Becoming a runner later in life has helped me gain some perspective on the joy of running that many lifetime runners don't have. Realizing that I am having the time of my life at this time in my life helps me understand how running has changed my life. Realizing that the worst day I've ever had as a runner was better than almost every day as a non-runner brings me closer to keeping my running fun.

After all, if it isn't fun, why do it? The most disciplined among us would have a difficult time accepting the challenges and frustrations of running just because the activity might add a little time to our lives somewhere down the road. No, focusing exclusively on the long-term benefits to the quality of our lives in the retirement years isn't going to make running fun for everyone.

For running to become a part of your life for the rest of your life, there has to be a way of finding a reward in the activity itself that is both immediate and sustained. Running has got to feel good *right now.* It must allow you to feel good in the afterglow of effort. And it's got to do that on a regular basis.

For me, running comes down to equal parts of inspiration, perspiration, dedication, and celebration. Each of these components is essential to a lifelong program of running, and each contributes to keeping running fun.

INSPIRATION

*I*nspiration grows out of our childlike need to constantly satisfy our curiosity. Children are curious about everything. There is no subject too mundane to be considered interesting by a child. From the mysteries of the universe to exactly what dog food tastes like, a child is filled with wonder.

It is only from wondering about a problem that one discovers the solution. Every discovery in history has begun with someone asking, "I wonder what would happen if . . . ?" Some of these wonderings, like when someone first said, "I wonder what would happen if we tried to land on the moon?" have produced monumental achievements. Others have been far more dubious, like when someone asked, "I wonder what would happen if we put peanut butter and jelly in the same jar?" From those moments of wonder come the inspiration to satisfy our curiosity.

I wondered what would happen if I became a runner. I might just as well have asked what would happen if I landed on the moon. I had no background, no experience, and, in fact, no interest in running since it stopped being fun at age nine or ten. But I began to wonder what would happen if I became a runner.

In my case, running became the means by which I would become a runner. It's hard, after all, to imagine being a runner and not running. But the inspiration for me came not in finding a way to run, but in finding a way to be a runner.

I found out that runners used certain kinds of shoes, ate certain kinds of foods, and wore certain kinds of clothes. I also learned that runners spoke their own language. It was the language of running.

As important as beginning to run was in satisfying my curiosity, so, too, was beginning to act and look more like a runner. If I was to find out what would happen if I became a runner, I was going to have to invest time and energy beyond the simple act of running. I was going to have to find out what being a runner meant, even when I wasn't running.

That fleeting curiosity about what being a runner would be like, that moment of inspiration, led to the sequence of curiosity, inspiration, and seeking solutions. I wondered what kind of running shoes I needed, what kind of running clothes to wear, what kind of training program to follow, where runners ran, and most important, how I would know if I was a runner.

From that first inspiration, I have continued to wonder about shoes and clothes and training. I've continued to try to satisfy my curiosity about running, about running better, and about myself as a runner.

PERSPIRATION

Running for your life means understanding enough about effort to know when enough is enough and how much is too much. It's easy to think about running as an activity that causes you to sweat. It's easy to look at that one element of running and believe that if you get the sweat glands going you're doing what needs to be done.

It's also very easy to get lost in the sweat. I worry when I see people running in rubber suits or heavy clothes that are designed to make them sweat. I know when I see them that it isn't the run that's important, it's the sweat. What is really important to them is the weight that the sweat is carrying off their bodies. Seeing the pounds disappear is the number-one goal of the run for them. Their joy is always short-lived.

To run for a lifetime, eventually one needs to understand how the body works and how the body processes effort. You can't hope or pretend that your body is different in design or operation. You've got to learn to work with your body to achieve your goals.

The training effect is real. So is the overtraining effect. The benefits of controlling effort are real. So are the risks in out-of-control enthusiasm. Knowing how to balance the level of effort with realistic outcomes is essential to a lifetime of running.

DEDICATION

We arrive at where we are in our lives one day at a time. If we wake up one morning and realize that we have drifted off course, we still have to make our way back one day at a time. There are no short cuts from where you are to where you want to be. You must be dedicated to the process of change, however slow that change may occur.

Running for life means being dedicated to the act of running as an expression of yourself. Runners run. It's as simple as that. But there are also times when runners *don't* run. The challenge is to be dedicated to being a runner both when you are and when you are not running.

Being a runner becomes integrated into every aspect of your life. In time, many of the choices about what to do or not to do become easier. You do whatever makes you feel most like a runner. You do what a runner would do. Some would argue that it's easiest to feel like a runner when you are running. From my perspective, that's not true at all. In fact, many times it is during the actual act of running that I feel the least like a runner.

When I'm running, I am all too aware of all the things that separate me from other runners. I know how slowly I am running, I know how awkward my stride looks. No, for me it is not while I'm running that I feel most like a runner.

It is in the daily moments of decision that I feel most dedicated to running and most like a runner. It is in the quiet time when I ask myself whether today is a day to run that I feel most like a runner. Even on those days when I decide not to run, I know that I am making that decision as a runner.

CELEBRATION

Running for life means learning to seize moments, large and small, for celebration. It means learning to find joy in the simplest revelations and the most marginal improvements. With practice, every run becomes an opportunity to celebrate, even if that means celebrating that the run is finally over.

Celebrating means being open to the unexpected. It may be the unexpected beauty of the day, the ease of your stride, or the quality of your effort. Any run can provoke a kind of spontaneous celebration.

Celebrating may occur in the company of others. There are days when your own running may not be what you wanted, but you can still share in the celebration of someone else's running. Those celebrations can be as dramatic as a race victory or as personal as watching a new runner complete his or her first race or achieve a new goal.

Together, inspiration, perspiration, dedication, and celebration form the foundation of a lifelong program of running. On the foundation of these each of us compiles the daily, weekly, and yearly reasons to run. On the foundation of these, each of us finds his own unique way of expressing himself as a runner.

I WAS AN OLD MAN THEN

One of the ways running expresses itself in my life is through my age. As a runner, the only birthdays that now matter are the ones that put me into a different age group. In a runner's world, there really isn't any difference between being forty-six and forty-nine years old.

Skipping birthdays is only one way in which running is slowing down my aging process. Through running, I'm actually getting younger. No, I'm not talking about the cardiovascular improvements. I am actually getting younger every year I run.

It helps that I was such an old man when I started running. I was well into my second marriage and third career when I took up running. My son was in college and my parents were at retirement age. And I was heading at top speed into middle age.

It's not that forty-three is all that old. In fact, I don't remember actually thinking that I was old. I just remember feeling that I no longer carried myself as a young person would. I wasn't old yet, but I knew I was headed in that direction.

By the time I reached forty-three, I was living an old man's life in an old man's body. Like most of my friends, I had begun dreaming old men's dreams. I thought about preparing for retirement, investing in an IRA, and whether I would have to work until I was seventy years old. I'm happy to report that I am much younger than that now.

My hopes and dreams have changed as dramatically as my body. I shed eighty pounds and thirty years at the same time. Not only do my clothes no longer fit, but I've had to get a whole new wardrobe of dreams. When I started running, I could count the years of accumulated excess around my waist like rings on a tree. The wear marks on my belt moved steadily outward. Inch by inch I was becoming more than I ever expected to be.

At the same time that my waist was expanding, my possibilities were shrinking. Every year there were fewer things I thought I could do, fewer places I thought I could go, and fewer people I thought I could grow up to be.

Unlike a tree, however, with each passing year I became softer on the outside but harder on the inside. The world around me came to matter less and less. The effort to care was becoming too much.

When I was an old man, I always seemed to be searching for something better. It didn't matter how much I had or how good it was; I was sure that there was something better out there. I traded in perfectly good cars in order to get what I thought would be better cars. They weren't. I gave up good jobs in the hope that the new job would be a better job. It wasn't.

Even my running started out that way. Almost as soon as I started running, I wanted to be better. If better meant running faster, I wanted to run faster. If better meant running farther, I wanted to run farther.

GETTING YOUNGER

As I have gotten younger, I've learned that most of what I thought was better was based on what someone else told me was better. I didn't question it when someone told me there was a better neighborhood, or a better watch, or a better restaurant. If it was perceived to be better, that's what I wanted.

Strangely, the younger I get, the more willing I am to trust my own judgment. I am willing to accept that things that are good for me may not be good at all for someone else. I'm also beginning to understand that, sometimes, I'm a better judge of better. The biggest revelation was realizing that I can't live every moment of my life as an adult. It's not necessarily better to be older. It's not necessarily better to act your age. So I don't.

Now that I'm younger, when I run, I run like I did as a child. I run because it makes me feel good. I run because it releases me from the strain of pretending to be an adult. I run because when I'm running I can forget how old I'm supposed to be and be as old as I want.

I've got to be careful, though. Sometimes I have to tell my non-running friends and even some of my adult running friends that I am training or doing a workout. They don't always understand if I start talking about running as a form of play. So I end up telling them about my perceived exertion. If they press me, I even talk about the intervals I run, or that I am trying to run at specific percentages of my maximum heart rate. It usually fools them, even though deep down I know that I'm just having fun.

I try really hard to maintain the façade of adulthood when I'm running. When non-runners see me, I quickly try to present an expression that is somewhere between euphoria and abject pain. That's what non-runners think we are experiencing. And I don't want them to be disappointed.

It get's real tricky for me when I see another runner approaching, though. First, I try to get that grim look of determination on my face. I check my watch, as if I've actually turned it on. I move my lips as though I am calculating some important piece of data about my run.

Then, as we pass each other, I give the traditional runner's grunt and wave. I try to sound particularly out of breath when I grunt. I've gotten pretty good at a kind of guttural gasp. Then, when I'm sure I'm safely out of sight, I relax and go back to having fun.

The biggest problem is at races. At races I have to try even harder to pretend that running isn't fun. At the start, I line up with a determined look on my face that says, "This is the day I'm going to test the limits of my abilities and the accuracy of my training." I try to get a decent stride going so that it looks like I'm planning to assault my PR at that distance. I put on my game face. But it doesn't last.

It doesn't take more than a mile or so before I settle into my childlike pace. Before long I am chatting with the other runners, encouraging those whom I pass, and congratulating those who pass me. I joke with the volunteers at the water tables explaining that, like James Bond, I want my sports drink shaken, not stirred. I have even been known to ask policemen if they've seen any really fast runners on the course before me.

For a long time I worried about what this meant. I was enjoying myself in the middle of a run or a race. I wondered if somehow I just wasn't getting it. I thought maybe I was missing some key element in being a runner. I had never seen anyone describe the kind of fun I was having in any training guide. No one had ever told me it was okay to have fun when you ran.

What really worried me, though, was that I couldn't resolve an apparent paradox. It seemed that the harder I worked at being a better runner, the more fun I had. The more disciplined I was about my training, the more carefully I planned my running and racing schedule, the better I got and the more fun I had. Training hard wasn't work, it was fun!

Running also provided me with some moments of absurdity. There were times when I was waddling around the university track doing quarter-mile repeats when the local high school track team showed up to practice. Being passed twice per lap is enough to make anyone laugh. But as slow and silly as I may have seemed to the high school track stars, the track workouts were making me faster.

The strangest activity, and one that I enjoy in spite of myself, is running on a treadmill like a caged gerbil. I can run on a treadmill for hours and not get bored. I just can't escape the fundamental silliness of it. How adult and rational can it be, I think, to spend an hour running on a rolling rubber mat?

The more I run like a child, the more childlike I am when I'm not running. When I was older, it would never have occurred to me to just have fun, without a purpose. Now that I am younger, I am much more inclined to episodes of pure foolishness. When I was older, I often was satisfied to be merely content. Now that I am younger, there are times when I am unapologetically happy. I don't know how much younger I can get, but I know that I will never allow myself to get as old as I used to be.

MOMENTS OF TRUTH

During our lives as runners, we face a moment of truth every time we put on our running shoes. In fact, it may be that the most important moment of truth comes just before we decide to put on our running shoes. In that powder flash of decision, we affirm our identities as runners.

Eventually, running for your life becomes the accumulation of thousands of seemingly meaningless and unrelated moments as a runner. Over time, it is the aggregate of all those dark mornings and cool evenings and weekend long runs that ultimately make us the runners we will become. Running for life is a choice we allow ourselves to make. The fate of the world, the safety of our loved ones, or the future of the planet hardly depends on our daily runs. The motivation to run doesn't come from a misguided notion that anything of significance hangs in the balance. We run simply because we are runners.

When I finally knew that I would run for the rest of my life, every run and every decision to run became another stone in the mosaic of my running life. Piece by piece I began fashioning a picture of myself as a runner that reflects not just who I am, but what I want to become. Little by little the pattern of myself as a runner is emerging.

Some stones in my mosaic glitter. For me they are not overall race wins or even age-group awards. They are the memories of extraordinary efforts. Other stones are a deeper hue. They represent the fear about an injury that might stop me from running or the quiet acknowledgment of an opportunity to excel stifled by my own insecurities.

For most of us who run for our lives, the stones in our mosaics are nondescript. They are the stones that signify the hundreds of days that we run when we don't have to. They symbolize all the rainy days and cold mornings and late nights that we run.

They are the stones of the extra miles we run for our souls, after we've trained our bodies. They represent all of the miles we've run to forgive and the miles we've run to forget, as well as the miles we have yet to run.

Day by day, moment by moment, we are adding to the mosaic of ourselves as runners. And every day that we are runners, not just on the days that we run, we are closer to completing ourselves.

Waddle on, friends.

INDEX